3/16

love, loss,
and
what we ate

love, loss, and what we ate

Padma Lakshmi

ecco

An Imprint of HarperCollins*Publishers*

HarperCollins books may be purchased for educational, business, or sales promotional use. For information please e-mail the Special Markets Department at SPsales@harpercollins.com.

FIRST EDITION

Designed by Suet Yee Chong

Library of Congress Cataloging-in-Publication Data has been applied for.

ISBN 978-0-06-220261-1 (hardcover)
ISBN 978-0-06-247398-1 (B&N signed edition)

16 17 18 19 20   OV/RRD   10 9 8 7 6 5 4 3 2 1

For TJF

The heart knows no pain sharper than love's arrow.

chapter 1

It was the end of summer and the end of a life as I had lived it. The year was 2007. Inside the Surrey Hotel, which I would come to call the "Sorry Hotel," then a musty residential place (much like the Chelsea Hotel, but without the artists), I sat on the floor with cardboard boxes towering all around me. These walls and floors cloaked in dusty beige and brown, with a linoleum- and Formica-laden kitchenette, would be my refuge—a place where the displaced, like me, put themselves.

One month earlier, I had finished moving out of my beautiful home: taking the last pictures off the walls, wrapping the last trinkets in tissue, and finally, nauseatingly, separating the wedding photos into two neat piles. Everything I had been carting from one stage of my life to another, to remind me of me, was in the boxes that surrounded me. And there were so many of them now, just days before my thirty-seventh birthday. But so little left of me. At the end of a marriage, no one wins. There is only anger, sorrow, guilt, emptiness, and defeat. Outside, it rained. There had been many rainy nights that summer.

I had been sitting, staring at nothing, for so long that my tailbone had started to throb. Far off, the muffled sound of a phone ringing and ringing finally penetrated my daze. As I rose to silence the phone, shifting my weight, I felt the sharp, sudden pull of surgical stitches on my abdomen. I reached out to steady myself against a box. As I did, it shifted. I heard the silky, scratchy rustle of cellophane against cardboard. Down tumbled dozens of dusty kumquats, from a bag that had been perched precariously on top of the stack. They were a gift from my worried mother, shipped from her garden in Los Angeles. When the avalanche stopped, my gaze focused on the bright, beautiful fruit, the orbs glowing orange against the dull backdrop of everything else. The man I had left was like that: he could illuminate any room, no matter how dim.

My future husband and I had met eight years earlier, in 1999, in the shadow of the Statue of Liberty. After my European modeling career had more or less come to a close in the late nineties, I embarked on a professional acting career in Italy. Starting in 1997, I also began to cohost an Italian television show called *Domenica In*. I was surprisingly busy with work, and after acting in two period miniseries in 1998, decided to build on what I hoped was a burgeoning career by moving back to L.A., where I had lived as a teenager. I came to New York frequently, too, as most of my friends and extended family lived there. I was finding my way again in the U.S. after spending most of my twenties in Europe. For the first time since college I was single. I dated some, but not seriously. Instead, I focused on auditions and on writing and then on promoting my first cookbook, *Easy Exotic: A Model's Low-Fat Recipes from Around the World*.

For my first role, I had to gain twenty pounds, which was a cinch and a pleasure. Best three months of my life. Losing the weight after filming ended, not so much. I wanted to do it in a healthy way. The regimen I came up with was not quite a diet. There was no deprivation involved, mainly because deprivation is miserable: the more brutal or austere the diet, the harder it is to keep. Instead, I tweaked recipes for my favorite foods from around the world in an attempt to excise calories but not flavor. And those recipes became *Easy Exotic.* I landed a publishing contract for the book largely because, well, everyone wants to know what a model eats.

Tina Brown, ex–*Vanity Fair* and *New Yorker* editor, had recently founded a new magazine, *Talk,* as well as a publishing imprint, Talk Books, in conjunction with Miramax Books. My book, left over from the previous Miramax list, was one of her first books. I doubt my silly little cookbook, closer to pamphlet than proper volume, was her first choice. But somehow, I was invited to the new magazine and book imprint's launch party, a Great Gatsbian affair on Liberty Island. It is still the best party I have ever been to, except of course for my own wedding, five years later.

On a balmy, beautiful August night, I came with a few friends, including my book editor (who would eventually become one of my bridesmaids). We all boarded the ferry and arrived at a fete lit by candles. Tina had invited such a strange and wonderful mix of people, a combination of the high-minded and the pop—a particularly glamorous herd of heads of state, cultural taste makers, movie stars, artists, models, writers, and other starstruck dilettantes like myself. After all, this was the woman who as editor in chief of *The New Yorker* had devoted (to jeers as well as to applause) an entire issue to fashion, starring writers like John Updike. She employed similar juxtapositions on the pages of *Vanity Fair,* too, and it had served both the magazine and her reputation well. It was what Tina was very good at. She brought really interesting people from the far ends of the cultural spectrum together. She enjoyed it. And she had the power to do it. It is a very important lesson in good hosting and curating that I still use today. This time, that room just happened to be all of Liberty Island. I found myself in an electric-turquoise Calypso slip dress (*so nineties*), laughing and dancing with the likes of Henry Kissinger, Todd Solondz, and

Madonna, excited about my first book and my new life back in America. Colorful fireworks lit the sky.

There was certainly magic at work that night. Typically, parties are the perfect setting for the spectator sport that is people-watching. But, whether intentionally or not, this party was so dimly lit that you couldn't quite see who the other guests were. There were low-wattage fairy lights strung about, powered by generators, but that was it. If you wanted to really experience the party and its luminaries, you had to dive in and walk around, get up close and personal. I found myself passing a very fair-skinned Indian man who looked familiar. We both turned somehow just in time as our eyes met. As we talked, I developed a hunch that this twinkly-eyed man with his arched eyebrows, salt-and-pepper beard, bald pate, and sharp nose might be Salman Rushdie. I was a teenager when the trouble had started, but even then I'd seen the images—I imagine most Indians had—of the man, our own Hemingway, whose life was under threat for his book *The Satanic Verses* and its supposed affront to Islam. His eminence was compounded by the controversy. But *this* man couldn't be him. He seemed to know all about me. He asked me about my life in Italy, my childhood in Madras. I decided he was probably some distant uncle.

At some point, he gave me what even a naïf like me recognized as a pickup line. "I've always been interested in Indian diaspora stories," he said, or something like that. "Perhaps we could talk about yours." I was game, I told him. We exchanged numbers. "Can you write your full name?" I asked, which must have seemed odd, but he said nothing and did. *Aha!* I thought, as I read the scrawl. It *is* him. I wasn't thinking very clearly but at least I'd have his autograph. This is how removed from my life this man was.

The next morning, I was in NoLIta, contemplating a Tracy Feith mustard-yellow scarf dress, when I got a call from a man with an Anglo-Indian accent. "Sorry, wrong number," the man said, and hung up. How strange, I thought as I bent over with the dress still half over my head in the tiny fitting room. I called back the number that now appeared on my nifty new cellular telephone. "Salman, is that you? Are you *crank calling* me?"

"Um, well yes, I think I just dialed the wrong number. But it didn't sound like you. Uh, what are you doing?" he asked, uncharacteristically fumbling for words.

"Trying on a dress. I think I like it."

"You should buy it," he said.

And I did.

So our telephonic relationship began. At first, I thought it strange that someone as important and, I assumed, busy as he must be had time to talk as often as we did. Little did I know that writers are incredibly gifted at finding ways *not* to write. I soon solved the mystery of how he'd known about my life. Several months prior, in the course of promoting his latest novel, he had been featured in the Italian magazine *Panorama*. Inside, there was a small profile of me—he'd read it and saved it.

I had just gotten my first American cell phone a month before we met and the novelty of being able to take him with me anywhere—the Santa Monica Pier or the farmers' market in West Hollywood—brought an intimacy to our calls. And a thrill, too. I described the world to him as I experienced it. I felt like a Bond girl with that phone pressed to my ear and that charming Anglo accent on the line. Years later I would see the film *Her,* by Spike Jonze, and identify with the main character's mounting feelings about a computer OS that he becomes emotionally attached to. What would my friends think of me, having this telephonic relationship with a married author almost a quarter of a century older than me and living in England with Special Branch security protection? The whole thing seemed surreal.

It's hard to explain now, but I fell in love with Salman over the phone. I was still in my twenties, and no one of his artistic or intellectual caliber had ever so much as crossed my path. He had such a mellifluous voice. Calm and mysterious, it gained an impish lilt just when he was telling you some juicy punch line. He had a wicked sense of humor and he seduced with his greatest weapon, his words. He knew how to construct the perfect compliments, too, layered with acute observations about me that seemed unimaginable coming from someone who'd been in my actual presence for mere minutes. He told me stories of his own childhood in Bombay, his early years in London. He confided in me and seemed interested in the most mundane and microscopic details of my new, lonely life in Los Angeles. He listened to stories of my childhood. He understood what it was like to be Indian in the West. He understood the awkwardness and melancholy of going back home, too. For the next three weeks we spoke two to three times daily.

In the soul-sucking intellectual desert that L.A. was for me at the time, I was starving for that kind of connection, and my future husband's phone calls were a nine-course meal airlifted in with iced champagne to boot. His attention, almost more than his charm, seduced me. Despite my small-potatoes cookbook deal and the occasional invite to a glitzy party, I was not exactly flying high in L.A. I had left a life of glamour and a dram of success as a model and, more recently, as an actress in Italy to return to the city of my adolescence. As a foreigner, I felt there was an implied limit to my career in Italy, where I would always be a curiosity. I wanted to try my hand in America before it was too late. I wanted to make the transition to more stimulating work before modeling decided it had had enough of me. Worse still, I was turning thirty in a little over a year, a milestone that in the business of appearance might as well be a gravestone.

That was the backdrop when he started calling. During a time when no one seemed interested in me in Los Angeles, a man came along who was, and not just any man. Once, he called as I stood at the sink eating a peach, the juice streaking down my arm. I picked up.

"Hi, Salman," I said. "Hold on for a second, I'm eating a peach."

"What color is it?" he asked.

Could I really be so inconsequential if Salman Rushdie wanted to know the color of my peach? It sounds silly in retrospect, but at the time, in the midst of a crisis of self-worth, I eagerly took up the fantastical notion that I had begun to inspire this great man.

Salman lived in London at the time, but he rented a place on Long Island every summer. He liked being in New York, where even during the fatwa he felt safe enough to enjoy the city without his typical security detail. After a few weeks, I was set to come to New York to make my first appearance on the Food Network to promote *Easy Exotic*. He told me he was soon returning to the city for work and asked if I'd like to have lunch. He said he was married sometime in the first week by saying he was here in the States with his "family." Nothing more. I knew damn well what he meant even though he had said it in the blandest way possible, but I didn't stop speaking to him, because I was incapable of giving up this new exhilarating presence in my life. Up to that point our connection had been only verbal, only telephonic. So it was easy to justify how I could keep speaking to him. Nonetheless, I didn't want to be that woman. I convinced myself that ours was a platonic relationship. Since no hanky-panky had gone on, I could continue my friendship with this man. I was powerless to refuse any contact from him whatsoever.

"I can't go with you to lunch," I said.

"It's just lunch."

Touché.

I proposed a stroll instead. It seemed simpler, more innocent, less fraught with potential for misunderstanding, less like a date. A walk, a stroll, could end at any time for any reason I could conjure up if needed. We were to meet at four o'clock in the afternoon on the steps of the Metropolitan Museum. He sat there waiting as I got out of the yellow cab, in my mustard-yellow dress. He wore his slightly rumpled look: a faded black T-shirt, baggy slacks, and a loose blue cotton jacket. We walked in Central Park, around and around the lake. The weather was perfectly sunny and pleasant. It was one of those rare late-summer afternoons when it's warm but not too hot. Sunlight streamed through swaying maple leaves. Families were trying to squeeze out the last drop of summer, picnicking on the grass. Teenagers were playing Frisbee. We heard snatches of music from street performers as we circled the lake, smelled the occasional whiff of pot smoke. We enjoyed Mister Softee cones and lingered until the lake glowed, until the sun sank behind the trees. I cannot remember what we talked about except that we never stopped talking. I suppose we spoke of everything and nothing, just happy to be speaking now while standing, finally, on the same ground together. I lost track of time but knew some hours had passed.

He was staying nearby at the Mark Hotel. I said I'd walk him there. Because neither of us wanted the day to end, we had a drink at the hotel bar. In an attempt to be cool, I ordered a single-malt Scotch on the rocks. I was so nervous that I drained my glass. I had dinner plans with friends nearby, so he walked me to the restaurant. Not thinking what it might imply, I invited him to come along and sit down with us. I just couldn't bear to say good-bye to him.

We fell into bed that night. At 3:00 a.m., I woke with a start. *I'm naked in a married man's bed.* I got dressed and skulked out of the Mark, feeling like a hussy. Once home, I showered, attempting to scrub away my shame. There were so many reasons we shouldn't be together. He was married, for one, with a young son. He lived in London. The ominous cloud of the fatwa hung over his head. He was twenty-three years my senior, old enough to be my father. I consoled myself by resolving that there was only one decision to make; the next step was too obvious to doubt. We would stop speaking. I would go back to my life and he to his. But he kept calling. And I kept answering. I could not resist him.

Speaking to his disembodied voice allowed me to convince myself that we were still two innocents. Our courtship already felt like a dream. His face had lit up television screens in India and around the world. Even before the trouble with Iran, he was considered a formidable writer and a great intellectual mind. Up close I had known only the weighty world of lingerie modeling. His gravitas was the spark that lit my attraction. He was everything I wasn't. He was a lot of what I wanted to be. He did not try to fit in. I had spent my career trying to be what other people wanted me to be, to embody whatever quality they felt was needed to sell jeans or bras or perfume. He had made a life of being different. I was totally taken by this man, and my admiration for him propelled me ever toward him. The fire burned because of his wit and charm and the connection between us. I had to admit, if only to myself, that this was not innocent, that now I had no platonic alibi to hide behind.

In him I had found a fellow wanderer, someone who knew what it was to always feel slightly displaced. In my case, I had spent years shuttling between India and the U.S., then later throughout Europe. He, too, was an Indian raised in the West. He understood my experience firsthand.

In L.A., I spent much of my time milling around commercial sets with teenagers. Many models don't finish high school. The girls were sweet, the conversation less than stimulating. I was intellectually curious and I wanted to be stimulated and challenged. I loved books. The important mentors in my life had valued learning. There was Mr. Henniger, my high school English teacher and Academic Olympiad coach, who threw end-of-the-year parties where you had to come dressed as a literary character. He came as Godot, a sign on his chest reading, "I'm here!" There was Michael Spingler, a French professor from my college and later, when I was a starving model in Paris, a savior who invited me into his home to share pots of beans and lardons with his friends—bookstore owners, poets, and authors. There was my grandfather, a hydro-engineer who retired only to get a law degree and become a practicing attorney, only to retire once more to become a tutor to college students studying math and science as well as the humanities. I was primed to value what Salman had to offer of himself, and it fed me so completely that I was blinded to everything else.

Salman wanted to see me once more that week before I went back to L.A. Again, he asked me to lunch, and again, I should have said no. This time, however, lunch seemed like the best option. Meeting in a public place meant we couldn't even hold hands. We met at Balthazar, the old-world SoHo brasserie, which in the late nineties was all the rage. Propriety be damned. My twenty-ninth birthday was approaching, and he handed me a copy of his latest book, *The Ground Beneath Her Feet.* On the title page, he had crossed out "her" and written "your," and signed it, "Love, Salman." As if this were not enough, he asked me what I would like as a present. As long as it wasn't a Maserati, he'd be happy to oblige. I'd known him then for less than thirty days. I searched my mind for something appropriate—it couldn't scream "mistress," and I couldn't exactly ask *Salman Rushdie* for a CD player. So I asked for a story. Sure, he said, he could easily dig up an unpublished piece in a drawer somewhere. No, I said, an original story. Something you write for me. The story synopsis that he wrote for Random House, and faxed to me, would eventually become *The Enchantress of Florence,* his ninth novel, finally published a year after our divorce.

Just three weeks had gone by since I'd first met him fleetingly on Liberty Island. We had indeed only been in each other's actual presence thrice. Yet I could no longer imagine a life without this man in it. I didn't know what had hit me. It was like living in a landlocked place all your life, and then one day seeing the ocean. And swimming in it. I had opened a door I didn't know existed. My heart leapt every time the phone rang. My heart began to sink every time a few hours went by and it didn't ring. Salman was a great talker. He could speak knowledgeably about anything, one minute enlightening you on an obscure eastern European author, then in the next moment speaking with fluency on Mexican music. He could use baseball stats to drive home a point about history. Even when I went out with friends in Los Angeles, or feigned interest in the dates I was still going on (what elaborate lengths we go to fool ourselves), the best part of the evening would be coming home and telling him all about it just as he woke in London. He could be erudite and serious. But he could also be sardonic. He was an equal-opportunity derider, poking fun at everything from poetry to pop culture. He often joked about poets, "Their words don't even go to the end of the page." I felt lofty by association, which buoyed my shaky confidence. I had achieved some measure of success in my industry in Europe, yes, but I was one of the only people in my family without a graduate degree. I had always felt conflicted about my work, at once proud of how far I had come and eager to prove that I had more to offer than a nice silhouette. I saw in him, even if I didn't admit it to myself at the time, the pathway to a life full of learning and growing.

Our relationship continued over the phone for several more weeks and I continued my life in L.A. as if nothing had changed. Only a year had passed since I'd moved back to the States after spending most of my twenties in Europe. My theater degree and lack of real job experience hung around my neck like a yoke. I had done two films in Italy, but I was hustling even to find an agent willing to take me on in Los Angeles. The book had done modestly well, and I soon got word it had won the 1999 Versailles World Cookbook Fair Award for Best First Book. They sent me a scrolled-up certificate with a very official gold seal on it. But no one knew or cared except my mother and my editor. My advance had long since been spent and it would be ages before I earned it out and saw any checks from book sales. It had been a few months since I'd published the book, and after the promotional tour, I returned to the slog of commercial castings and the loneliness of California, the isolation chamber of my mom's '86 Nissan Stanza. This was the same car I had learned to drive in at sixteen.

Regardless of all I had seen and done, in college and abroad in Milan and Paris as a model, as an actress and TV host, I suddenly didn't feel like I had come very far from those high school days. Los Angeles would have this effect on me until years and years later.

That November Salman's latest novel was to be published in French and he would be going to Paris to celebrate. "Come with me," he said. "I'll send you a ticket." I had to say yes, yes to Paris, to an escape from L.A. And yes to him. I couldn't refuse the adventure.

I'll admit I applied very little rational thought to the decision to go. I didn't think of what accepting the invitation might mean. People are so strange, aren't we? This man invited me to Paris. We'd spent so many nights baring our souls on the phone. We'd slept together once—months ago, but still. And yet I insisted that we stay in separate hotel rooms. God forbid a rendezvous in the City of Love with a married man have a whiff of impropriety.

The trip lasted about four days and immediately introduced me to the realities of the fatwa. When I arrived at the hotel, Salman and I managed a brief hello before I was introduced to the officers assigned by the French government to his protection. The head of security in Paris was a stocky black man with a shaved head, who looked stern and terrifying until he smiled. He was a teddy bear and comforted me with his warm presence. "*Je suis le Kojak negre,*" he told me when I asked his name, flashing that disarming grin, and a lollipop! *Just call me the black Kojak.*

There was an official dinner hosted by the English ambassador and a reading of Salman's work by the French actress Marie-France Pisier. I met Salman's publisher, Ivan Nabokov, Vladimir's grandson. We even went to visit my old professor and mentor, Michael Spingler, who still lived in the same apartment on Rue d'Alésia where I had spent so many happy evenings with his family.

Throughout the trip, my separate hotel room stayed empty except for my bags, my bedsheets unrumpled. But I suppose it was good to have it there in case the spell was broken somehow, now that we were actually in each other's physical presence for more than a few hours at a time. Or, perhaps, what if his wife suddenly showed up? I was aware that I was involved in something indecent, otherwise why would I have asked for the room in the first place? I had become one of those women you read about and cannot imagine being. My morality and sense of right were eroded by the allure of this man's ardor and attention. That I could burn one day for the sin of choosing adventure over decency did not deter me from running toward that adventure. I cannot remember a distinct moment when I made the decision to offer myself to this married man, a thing that until it happened would have been unthinkable to me. I suppose drowning my inhibitions in Scotch at the Mark Hotel in August had allowed me to break the glass of propriety, but now there was little will left in me to put a halt to things, to say no to the best thing that had ever happened to me. I still thought we'd soon go back to our separate and very different lives. But for those four days, I wanted to savor every second of my unexpected and fantastical jaunt, an adulterous Cinderella not wanting the clock to strike twelve.

That December, I went back to India, as I almost always do over Christmas. At my grandmother's house, between meals and temple visits, I gave myself a crash course in Rushdie. I couldn't get enough. I read *The Moor's Last Sigh*, set in Kerala, my family's ancestral home; *Midnight's Children*, a story of India's independence told through a writer who is involved with a cook named Padma and another girl later known as Parvati (my middle name); *Shame*; and *The Ground Beneath Her Feet*. I had read some of *The Satanic Verses* when I was young, and tried again. Every time he'd call, I'd recount what I'd just finished reading. It was great fun being able to ask the author to clarify or expand on any given page on any given day. I began to fall in love with his writing, too.

Due in part to his presence in my life, I had begun to grow as a person. I spent the night of the millennial New Year at an orphanage in Chennai (née Madras), cooking for the children there and playing until we fell asleep before midnight. I suppose I had to find a way to cleanse my soul as well.

On one of the first few times we spoke in the new year, Salman had an announcement. By phone he reported that he had asked his wife for a divorce. As hard as it might be to believe, this development was a shock to me. I don't know what I expected from our relationship, but I had not expected that. We had never discussed our future. We had never discussed the idea of his divorcing his wife. My reaction was a fully emulsified mixture of shock and guilt. I didn't want to be responsible for breaking up a little boy's family. I didn't get it. We'd spent a total of less than two weeks together (if you added up New York, Paris, and a trip he made that winter to L.A.) and he was leaving his wife? I insisted he not divorce his wife on my account. He assured me again and again that the marriage had been over before we met. We decided to keep things between us as they were, to not make any sudden moves.

But my intentions and worries proved no match for my affection. I still scurried to the phone when I thought a call was from him. I was young, starstruck, and lovestruck, and after a few months, we started making plans. I spent time traveling to and from L.A. and Salman went to his usual award ceremonies, symposiums, readings, and the like. I often came along. I joined him in Amsterdam for the Boekenbal, the ball that launched Dutch Book Week, when he was the first foreigner they ever honored. I still look at photos of that ball to remember the couple we once made: He in his tux and gray beard, which still had a streak of black near the chin. Me, in a sleeveless red gown and little diamond earrings, which I had bought years before during my early modeling days, my first-ever extravagant purchase. ("Seven hundred dollars!" my mother had yelped when I told her.) We looked so in love. Few people could spend time with us without feeling our charge.

I was eager to leave L.A. and had wanted to move back to New York. He, too, loved the city, and so it was decided. We moved in together in the spring of 2000. We rented a gorgeous brownstone on the Upper West Side with four floors, including a grand dining room dominated by an ornately carved wooden fireplace. The dining room had a little bay window that looked onto the back garden. We sublet this place for six months. This was the house in which my husband would write *Fury*. Our landlords lived upstate on a farm that supplied many of the city's finest restaurants. Every now and then, they'd send us a crate of vegetables—leeks and zucchini, carrots and tomatoes. I remember making a lot of ratatouille that summer.

My American television career began to take off. In the course of my book tour for *Easy Exotic*, I'd appeared on the Food Network a couple of times, and that had led to a development deal the following spring just as soon as we had moved in together. I would join *Melting Pot*, a series that aired every day at the same hour, each episode featuring a different pair of tag-team chefs representing a particular world cuisine.

There was Team Latino with Aarón Sánchez and Alex García. There was Team Mediterranean with Rocco DiSpirito and Michelle Bernstein. Michael Symon and another chef had the midweek eastern European slot. There was Caribbean cooking and soul food from the South. And then on Fridays there was me: Team, well, International Brown, I guess. The show was called *Padma's Passport*. Oddly, I had no cohost. And of course, I wasn't a chef, but a home cook. It was the first time—but far from the last—that I would feel completely out of my depth in the food world. Meanwhile, I still occasionally auditioned for parts in L.A. and New York. I played a bitchy, talentless pop singer named "Sylk" in Mariah Carey's *Glitter*. I played a kidnapped princess on *Star Trek: Enter-*

prise. Nothing groundbreaking, but I was having fun and happy to be working.

The next few years were, for the most part, blissful. I was in love. I soon was living in a beautiful house, which Salman bought and which I renovated. I trawled Simon's Hardware for knobs and handles and hired contractors. We restored the brownstone from four apartments to its original glory as a Gilded Age single-family home. When we were together in New York, even before we moved out of our sublet, we had our daily routine. Salman typically woke before I did. He'd make me green tea with honey and buttered toast and sweetly set it on my bedside table. I'd go to the gym, shower, then go to auditions or jobs or sit at a stool in the kitchen with my laptop, cooking and reading in preparation for my show. I overthought the process, researching cardamom and rehearsing the dozens of facts I'd learned so I would be armed with enough things to say on camera. I was learning on the job and until then had only my experience on Italian television to go by. I'd do my own work until I knew Salman's daily writing session was almost over, then I'd bound up the stairs to the third floor, where his office was, all the while thrilled that I lived in New York City. In a house. With a staircase.

I'd poke my head into his office and find his lap. Occasionally, he'd show me drafts of his work—an article for *The New Yorker,* an op-ed for *The Guardian*—and I'd pore over each one, trying to impress him with my thoughtful feedback. He ultimately made it clear that anything but my gushing approval would be ignored. But I didn't mind. He was the writer, after all.

One summer, we were walking together in the middle of Central Park when it suddenly started to rain. The clouds spilled sheets of water on us, and we took shelter under a tree. I was tugging at his arm, trying to pull him back out into the downpour, because after growing up on Bollywood rain sequences, the notion seemed quite romantic to me. He wouldn't budge, muttering about not wanting to turn his clothes into a soppy mess. I just laughed then. When you're in love, such differences of opinion seem beguiling.

At my most ardent, I sought to please and charm him, by preparing his favorite foods, decorating our home, looking my best, and telling him funny stories that I had rehearsed in my head on the way home to him. We had countless dinner parties for our friends, and I tried to create evenings that would please everyone, but particularly him. I loved hearing him hold forth from the head of the table, telling his layered stories as I flitted in and out of our kitchen barefoot. My feet throbbed as we lay in bed, satiated after those long evenings, reliving what funny things everyone had said and done as we fell asleep in each other's arms. We had our own patois, a jumble of East and West, a language of love and humor for comparing notes on the world.

Early on, I was both entranced and terror-stricken by his friends. I didn't realize that authors, like basketball players, hung out together. His friends were literary giants like Susan Sontag, Peter Carey, and Don DeLillo. Dropped in the middle of these people, I was unsure of myself and daunted by what he had said about them. I loved talking about books, but I was in constant fear that my English-lit-class knowledge would extinguish itself midsentence. And so I would sometimes retreat to the kitchen, where I could relish our guests and their stories from a safe distance. At the table, among others, were Don and his wife; Paul Auster and his second wife, Siri Hustvedt, herself an accomplished writer; their daughter, Sophie, barely a teenager; and Susan Sontag.

My insecurity at meeting Salman's friends revealed itself mostly in my cooking. My strategy for overcoming feelings of inferiority was to keep my hands busy, to cook and bring drinks and clear plates. For our first dinner party in our Upper West Side sublet, I planned a simple Indian menu. Our food is more regional than most Westerners realize, and I wanted to show the nuances of flavor from both my South Indian roots and Salman's northern Kashmiri ancestry. I had perused a cookbook written years ago by Salman's sister and noted that as kids they loved chicken—their father would complain about how much Salman and his sisters wanted to eat it all the time. The first four recipes all had yogurt in them. It was common for North Indian and especially Kashmiri dishes to have yogurt or cream, so I made a creamy chicken curry with mint from my first cookbook named after my uncle Chidambaram. The recipe called for a healthy dose of fiery dried red chilies, as well as garam masala, a North Indian spice blend of freshly dry-roasted and ground spices such as cinnamon, coriander seed, cardamom, and cumin.

I wanted Salman to feel not just at home, but like he was *back home,* where we were from. It was how he made me feel. I could not be his first wife (or his second or third for that matter). Indeed, because of our age difference, I could not experience many of his firsts with him. But I could, with my cooking, take him back home, to a sweet, idyllic place and time, back to those smells of childhood and India. I wanted him to feel that with me, he *was* finally home.

I found a heavy cast-iron pan, heaved it up onto the stove, and began to roast the whole spices and chilies together. I tossed around the coriander seeds and cinnamon twigs, scraping the pan with my metal spatula as I raked them back and forth. My eyes began to burn and tear as the spices released their oils. The aroma of those spices I hoped would be carried upstairs to his workroom, where he sat writing. I ground them up in an old Vitamix and wondered if our landlords would ever get the smell out of the machine. I doubted the sweet patrician kitchen with eyelet curtains and Betty Crocker décor had ever been assaulted with such smells. I made a mental note to soak the inside of the flask with lemon juice.

I made white beans with tomatoes and *amchur,* or dried green mango powder. The plump, round pink tomatoes here in the U.S. tasted bland

and watery to me most of the year. I took to adding a pinch of palm sugar and green mango powder to duplicate the sweet and sour notes in the less good-looking but delicious tomatoes from back home. I used a whole stick of butter to fry the ginger and red onions in the wok, before adding the rest of the ingredients. There was a street-food stew we ate with fluffy white bread buns as children called *pav bhaji*. I remembered having it first in Pune when I went to visit my aunt Neela after her marriage. There would be a semicircle of scooters and motorcycles gathered around a man with a huge black iron griddle about three feet across. Here the various vegetables would be bubbling away with tomato and ginger, a ton of not ghee, but Amul butter. Whole bricks would be buried in the hot stew, which got darker and darker as night set in. The tangy mix of ginger and dried green mango, fat and spices, bathed the soft, buttery white beans in just enough heat.

I made delicate lemon rice, common in our southern state of Tamil Nadu. Mustard seeds and curry leaves (sent from my mother's garden in Los Angeles), fresh serrano chilies, and white gram lentils were fried in hot oil with turmeric and cashews. That hot oil was mixed into the rice with fresh lemon juice and kosher salt. The bright-yellow hue would look stunning at the table. And to cool things off, I made *raita*, a yogurt-and-cucumber relish.

I kept my hands a little too busy—I cooked three times the amount I should have. We didn't even have room in the fridge for the leftover lemon rice and *raita*, the curried chicken with cream, or the white beans. But luckily, everyone seemed to enjoy the meal. Beautiful young Sophie proclaimed she liked the spread and would be happy to take much of it home, which a few of the guests did.

It helped, too, that I cooked. Who doesn't like the cook? My favorite among the guests was Don. I often found myself, at dinner parties and Thanksgivings, sitting with him. He spoke to me, as he always seemed to, softly and with great care. The opposite of pretentious, he spoke about his work, if at all, as a plumber might about installing pipes. Generously, he treated me like a peer. My favorites aside, I appreciated them all for their kindness toward me. If they were judging me, they never let on. For all of Salman's warnings that there was "good Susan and bad Susan," Ms. Sontag was always a pussycat.

My relationship wasn't all glamour and high-minded discussion, of course—and thank goodness. Early on, acquaintances would ask me breathlessly, "So does he just walk around being brilliant all the time?"

"Yes," I'd say. "I keep a notebook on me at all times to record every word."

"Wow, what did he say last night?"

"He told me to stop hogging the sheets."

chapter 2

By 2001, I had begun writing for magazines: first *Vogue*, then a style column in *Harper's Bazaar*, and a regular stint on food and fashion at the *New York Times* syndicate. I was still doing occasional modeling jobs here and there, but I began to enjoy the writing much more. That is to say, I enjoyed having written, once the piece was done. I still had serious insecurities as a writer, which being published did nothing to assuage. I was lucky in that Glenda Bailey of *Harper's* and Gloria Anderson at the *Times* pretty much left me to write about whatever interested me. I began by doing a piece for Anna Wintour on the scar on my arm, but I was terrified of writing it. Here, my future husband was extremely supportive and edited the piece before it went to *Vogue*. Having him upstairs in his office while I was down in the basement writing was daunting. But if I really got in a jam, it was also helpful—except that he knew little about fashion and had little patience for being interrupted. But he damn well did know how to write.

The series on the Food Network did not get renewed after the first season. I did land a gig hosting a couple of documentaries called *Planet Food* for the network and for Discovery International. A sort of light precursor to Anthony Bourdain's *No Reservations* (but with better hair!), it involved my traveling to a country and getting to know its people through their food. They were hard shoots, but I was totally in my element. I loved nothing more than spelunking around a place and tasting my way through it. I had done as much throughout my modeling career anyway. All those years of traveling to shoot French bras in Bali and Scottish sweaters in the Seychelles led me to taste and experience the world in a way I would have never been able to otherwise.

Because I had started modeling later than most, after my bachelor's degree, I was able to appreciate it more. At the end of those many trips, my suitcase was jam-packed with strange spices and sauces, seeds and twigs. I would use these in my own kitchen back in Milan, Paris, or New York to try to re-create what I had tasted in those various corners of the planet. Coming from India and spending what seemed like most of my upbringing in the kitchens of my grandmother, mother, and various aunts (that's where all the action was, after all), I valued and took a keen interest in spices. Living and cooking in Europe during my twenties taught me for the first time about French technique. And the modeling jaunts afforded me the possibility to learn how people ate in other parts of the world. But I was just a good cook with a bottomless curiosity about food. I had never in my life entertained the idea of a career in the culinary arts in any form until the Food Network thought I was capable of one. I still wasn't sure they were right. I would have never even thought of publishing that first cookbook, but my publisher, who suggested the idea, thought there was a marketing hook, banking on our culture's curiosity about models and their diets.

The acting was slow going; my degree in theater mattered little. I would audition for parts in films and TV while still writing and modeling. I'd get a few bites or at least callbacks. Often I heard that they liked me but just "weren't going ethnic with this role." When it finally came out,

Glitter was panned. The transition out of modeling and into a new career was a very haphazard and gradual one. I had to look hard at where my professional life was going and decide to be open to whatever work there was. My modeling career had been born of financial necessity, and then pursued because I had become easily accustomed to the lifestyle and, of course, the money. I had been able to pay off my college loans before many of my peers even settled into their first jobs or careers. But I felt some measure of self-loathing and deep insecurity for being in a profession that didn't engage my mind, that seemed to be due to no accomplishment of my own but rather to the alchemy of the genes endowed to me by my parents. I wasn't feeling guilty or bothered enough, however, to do something about it until the flow of work slowed down. My schedule also made it easy for me to travel around the globe with Salman for awards, literary festivals, and red carpets, but it was unpredictable and work came in waves. It was hard to plan dinners with friends and then have to cancel them at the last minute because some shoot or modeling job came up. And bookers don't eagerly continue to push for work for capricious girls with catalog and ad clients. I was luckier than many of my colleagues making the same transition, because I had a roof over my head. Still, I was anxious to make something of myself beyond modeling and prove my worth to my family back in India. I knew they were happy for me. My modeling had brought me much financial success, and also brought me home to India more often. But I am not sure if I could call what they felt about my work "pride." The thing that gave me the most satisfaction was cooking. In the kitchen I felt happy and confident.

Eventually, I got around to signing another contract with my publisher, who had been asking for a second cookbook for quite some time. This was right before my marriage to Salman. I had been tinkering with recipes for a few years, but my other writing always took me away, as did those intermittent auditions. I would stop everything I was doing to study my lines or finish an article on deadline. I also had, of course, to sit home on these occasions instead of accompanying my future husband to the many events he developed an appetite for attending. Salman's movements had been so extremely curtailed and limited by the fatwa and the entailed security issues that now that he was free—or freer—to go about his business, I found he was making up for lost time. Who could blame him?

At first it was fun going to all those events. I met many wonderful people I would have never had occasion to come across. I was modeling, acting, writing, and now about to embark on getting another book published. I was also trying to develop another show on food. It became difficult to manage it all. When I was cooking, I felt the hours slip by. I was never so happy as when barefoot in the kitchen with my hands sticky and my hair smelling slightly of grease. My schedule was erratic and unpredictable. It was a bummer to stop what I was doing in the kitchen, shower, and go to audition for a part that I knew I probably wouldn't get. I should have been happy to have the audition. Wasn't it what I wanted? Hadn't I studied for a chance to do precisely this?

My acting work was picking up: I had just been cast as Princess Bithia in ABC television's new version of *The Ten Commandments*, which meant I would be away for five weeks in Morocco filming. Salman grumbled about my being away that long. Coming to visit me in a Muslim country was not a possibility. Indeed, the producers hired two security officers to accompany me twenty-four hours a day, the whole time I was there. I felt embarrassed because I was the only actor who needed this precaution due to my personal life. But I was relieved that the producers were willing to hire me in spite of this additional expense.

I still wanted to find a way to combine being in front of the camera with my love of all things culinary. I wanted to do another show about food and culture. I had loved doing *Padma's Passport*, but I didn't want to do another how-to show. I took to hosting *Planet Food* like a duck to water and found I was actually pretty good at it. I had a glorious time doing that show. Being thrown on Italian television when I was at the tail end of my modeling days in Italy as part of the cast of *Domenica In* taught me much about hosting. You had to be quick-witted and ready for anything. You had to gauge the set and your guests and adjust accordingly. The adrenaline rush of having no script and being on live TV suited me well. I learned so much on *Domenica In* that I still use today. I wanted to go back to TV, as a host, and do another show on food. I met an executive at the E! network in L.A. who suggested I meet with her friend in New York at Bravo. I was an avid watcher of their show *Inside the Actors Studio,* and I knew they had had great success with *Queer Eye for the Straight Guy.* So I went up to 30 Rockefeller Center to see Bravo's president, Lauren Zalaznick. She and her vice president Frances Berwick listened intently to my pitch. My idea felt too narrow and highbrow for them; they needed something broader with more mass appeal. But they did want to do something in the food space. And to that end, they were developing a food competition show and wondered if I would be part of it.

I would meet with Andy Cohen and Dave Serwatka of Bravo and have numerous long conversations with Shauna Minoprio, the show's first executive producer. At first skeptical of the idea of reality television (I tended to watch PBS and the History Channel), I was impressed by how these people wanted to turn food into a serious competition. Shauna referenced the old seventies show *Master Chef* in England, which I had seen years back and liked. She spoke passionately about wanting the new show to be a proper professional competition rather than some bonhomous how-to show about who could make the best Bundt cake. She loved Julia Child but had no interest in adding to the pile of imitators already on TV. They had researched the food world and even gotten Tom Colicchio of Gramercy Tavern fame as a head judge and a woman named Gail Simmons of *Food & Wine* magazine to participate. I was excited to be part of the show. Little did I know that I would spend the next decade with these folks.

In the meantime I was still reading for parts both here in America and in London. We spent half our time in the UK because of my husband's children. I felt the self-induced pressure of making something out of myself and I wasn't going to wait for these TV people to get their ducks in a row. I was still writing for magazines but I could do that anywhere, and it actually helped to be in Europe during the fashion shows. The writing also made me more portable, so it was easier to travel with Salman. I noticed he would get grumpy if my schedule conflicted with his, and lately I seemed to always be in the wrong place at the wrong time.

I found it hard to keep all these balls in the air. Salman and I had married in the spring of 2004, and I had hoped that this would bring a sense of calm and additional security to our relationship. That we would settle somehow into a rhythm of work and life. But I was never there enough for him. I was struggling to keep him happy while still pursuing all the things I thought would lead to a life not reliant on modeling lingerie or selling shampoo—or on my husband, for that matter. If I got a callback, I was happy, but then I'd have to break it to my husband that I couldn't leave with him on one of his upcoming trips to Austria or Brazil. If I told my agent I couldn't go to the callback, my agent (who had been hard to get in the first place) would think I was crazy.

By the time Bravo was ready to shoot the food show, I had signed on to do a miniseries for British television called *Sharpe's Challenge* with an actor from the *Lord of the Rings* film trilogy named Sean Bean. It was a real bodice-heaver, a period piece set in India during the British Raj. We were to be on location for several weeks, this time in Jaipur, Rajasthan. And I, of course, was to play the local evil queen. Fantastic, I thought. Now we're getting somewhere. Andy Cohen, the programming head of Bravo, called, and I had to tell the network I couldn't do the food show.

On the other hand, I had done two miniseries in the same year. I finally felt like my career was taking shape and taking a permanent turn away from modeling.

My culinary ambitions would have to wait. But I watched the first season of *Top Chef* when it came out, and I thought it had some great elements. For the first time, I heard haute cuisine and fine dining being discussed on TV as they were in real life, analyzed matter-of-factly and without pretense. I was frankly surprised it wasn't too inside baseball for most viewers. But I loved what Bravo and the production company Magical Elves had done. They had made the rarefied world of gourmands and Michelin-starred chefs approachable and understandable to those in the audience who weren't necessarily food lovers, or "foodies," as they would come to be called.

Then one day, several months later, I got a call from Andy Cohen again. "Are you free *now*?" he asked. They were green-lighting the show for a second season, and while the ratings were modestly good, they were going to make changes and put a lot more resources behind it. *Top Chef* would become the thing most Americans would know me from. I had no idea how long it would last or what it would mean. I had done live television in Italy and I liked hosting. I had wanted to do some type of work around food. I was still working on my second cookbook, and the show could definitely give it a boost. It seemed like fun. Who wouldn't want to sit around eating delicious food and talking about it all day?

My first season, we shot in Los Angeles. Luckily, my husband also had to be in L.A. for part of it and so could visit. It was daunting how many hours it took to shoot a one-hour program. I was used to live TV and we'd just basically flown by the seat of our pants on the Food Network. Here we did, too, but the "hurry up and wait" of it all was insane. Since then we've gotten much better at streamlining the show, but things can still take a while. We were shooting at UCLA and I remember thinking how nice it was that my husband could finally come to see me working. But watching a TV show being made isn't all it's cracked up to be, and he soon got bored and went back to the hotel.

Things were going really well for me professionally and I started feeling better about myself. Just as I was convinced my days appearing in magazines were over, *Newsweek* called to tell me they wanted to put me on their cover to go with a story about the "New India." I was totally thrilled and couldn't believe it. I got off the phone and ran upstairs to tell Salman. He was at his desk and as usual I crawled up onto his lap. The moment I looked into his face and uttered the news, some knee-jerk reaction inside me braced for his reply. Lately, anytime I had some good news about my professional life, it seemed to interfere somehow with us. He just said, "That's great, I'm happy for you. The only time *Newsweek* put me on their cover was when someone was trying to put a bullet in my head." I didn't know how to react. I didn't want to anger him by saying the wrong thing or overreacting. I just wanted him to be proud of me, for us to savor this moment together.

I hoped he was indeed glad for me, if only because of how happy it made me. He seemed irked in some barely perceptible way. Lately, we hadn't been getting along as well. I couldn't shake the feeling I wasn't meeting his expectations as a wife. Indeed, at times he had told me as much. And I began to replace my insecurity about work with insecurity about my marriage.

On top of this discord, my menstrual cramps had worsened more and more over the last few years. I had always had pain every month and was used to taking a lot of pain medication during that time, but recently I felt the effects longer and more severely. During these times, I did not want to make love or be intimate in any way, and I actually found it hard to sleep because of my chronic pain. Plus, I was a light sleeper and my husband snored, and that had gotten worse over the years, too.

I had been in pain for more than two decades. It had started on the morning of my thirteenth birthday with my first menses. The dark liquid, thick and oozing from me, heralded almost immediately a lifelong companion—cramping, pain, a numbing ache. It wasn't very strong at first. I was distracted from the onslaught of my burgeoning womanhood. The hair that grew between my legs and in my armpits, the newly puffy nipples, and a general awkwardness were as difficult to accept. Pain had not been totally unexpected anyway. My own mother had primed me for what lay ahead. "Some girls get it, and some girls don't. It's just our lot in life, part of being a woman," she said. I had seen her miss work because of her own monthly pain, seen her take pills and lie with heating pads and hot-water bottles. Throughout my adolescence the pain grew, in intensity and duration, as did the flow of blood from my deepest insides. In college at Clark University, I begged my roommate to drive to the all-night pharmacy on Route 9 in Shrewsbury at midnight when I needed to retrieve more pain medication the doctor had prescribed. I became moody during what seemed like a third of the month and wondered if I would suffer from intermittent bouts of depression, as my mother had started to during my high school years.

Soon I began to have pain not only during that one week in the month I bled, but also while ovulating. I could tell which ovary produced the egg to be expelled that month just by where the pain emanated from. Along with cramping, bloating, and a general achy malaise, I began to feel my whole pelvis go numb. And at times, I also had lower back pain, and a pain that could shoot down one leg. I suffered severe nausea and headaches, too, though I could not tell if they were from my period or from the various pharmaceuticals I took to quell what was blandly referred to as menstrual "discomfort" or dysmenorrhea. No doctor seemed to know why. Nothing had eased my condition for long.

One day, nine months before Salman and I separated, I was at a studio, shooting the photos for my second cookbook. There's a photo of me by a window, looking out onto the Bowery. In it, I look contemplative and happy, pretty. In the real world, I was realizing I had started bleeding, and was hoping against hope the blood wouldn't leak through my underwear and onto my clothing. I hadn't brought tampons—I was two weeks into my cycle—so that afternoon, I stuffed my underwear with tissue.

My family doctor was already worried. He knew I'd had problems connected with my period and sent me to see a specialist on the Upper East Side. The day of the appointment was a hectic one. I rose at five that October morning to do an early cooking segment on the *Today* show. The day included, among other things, a work lunch, meetings with my editor and a group of buyers about the release of my new cookbook, and an early dinner at Bergdorf Goodman, where my publisher's wife was launching her evening dress collection. I squeezed in my appointment just after running home to change and just before the dinner.

When I hailed the cab to the doctor's office, I had on a shiny, strapless Marchesa cocktail dress embroidered with large cranes and flowers in gold, green, and magenta thread. The birds' wings and eyes twinkled with little sequins. My TV makeup from the morning had faded nicely, and in the car I touched up my lipstick so I would be ready to dash to the dinner afterward.

In the office, I took a seat across from the doctor at his desk, feeling silly for being so overdressed. The doctor, Tamer Seckin, came in and asked me a series of very thorough questions, almost too personal, even for a medical doctor. "How are your sexual relations with your husband?" "Has your libido dwindled over the years you have been together?" (Doesn't everyone's?) "What is your emotional and mental state during the week of your period?" "Do you have gas, or constipation?" "Do you ever argue about sex?" "Do your bra and pant sizes change within a month?" "Do you become irritable inexplicably?" "Have your period and the surrounding symptoms ever been an issue in your professional or home life?" "Do you feel understood?" I was taken aback.

He asked me to don a papery gown and meet him in the exam room. When I stripped down, I noticed deep red grooves imprinted on my torso from the dress's corset. In my effort to multitask the day, I hadn't thought things through. I wondered if he would think me so superficial that I was willing to constrict myself in the garment so extremely in order to look good. But surely he had seen a corset or two in his time?

I felt embarrassed in front of this doctor and not solely because of my nakedness, yet I didn't completely understand why. The nurse held my hand, and Dr. Seckin wielded what I learned later was a pediatric speculum. I squeezed her hand to fight the pain. He performed two exams, one that I had never had before. He did a rectal exam. No one who had ever examined me in all my thirty-six years had ever performed that exam. No gynecologist had ever been so invasive, physically or otherwise. After he had finished, he asked me to get dressed and meet him in his office. The clock above his head read 6:52 p.m. I had a dinner to get to.

"Will it take long, doctor?" I asked.

"Yes, Ms. Lakshmi, it might."

Sonograms and speculums can see beyond even the most sincere smile, the most glamorous cocktail dress. Sitting across from Dr. Seckin, I heard the word "endometriosis" for the first time. Over the course of the last twenty years, I had dutifully gone for checkups. I had seen doctors and specifically gynecologists of both sexes in various countries around the world. All of them were fine with prescribing pain pills for regular consumption, and reiterated what my mother had said when I first found out about the atrocities my body was capable of in the name of womanhood. Yes, for some women, it's a lifelong curse, they echoed. No one indicated that what was happening was serious, or damaging long-term, or anything like that. Some doctors thought I was exaggerating. Others became irate, including a woman who insisted that it couldn't hurt *that* much while she pushed her cold metal speculum inside me. I flinched, wincing in pain. One doctor actually smoked during the exam in Milan. I minded the smoker much less, especially since he at least put me on birth control, which did help for a time during my twenties.

I had quit using birth control a few months after my husband and I first moved in together, just around my turning thirty. Spending my twenties under the influence of hormones was enough and I could see the side effects taking their toll on my skin. I had also spent most of that time as a smoker and that had preyed on my mind, too. Now at the age of thirty-six, my body, unbeknownst to me, had been going full tilt for six years, producing excess tissue it could not expel at a much more rapid rate than in my twenties, when I was on contraceptive hormones to suppress the disease and its effects.

A healthy female body, Seckin explained, expels uterine lining during menstruation. Not so in the case of a woman who has endometriosis. Instead, the tissue pools in the body's reproductive cul-de-sac. The body then reabsorbs the lining, which grows. But the lining is no mere plasma or scar tissue; it has glands and responds to hormones—forming layer upon layer in the uterus, a new one each month that spills out into the peritoneum, or lower abdomen. It can pool outside the uterus and attach itself to all the internal organs of a woman with the condition, preventing normal functioning of those organs. It can choke her reproductive system, as weeds in a healthy garden can take down the tallest of shrubs. It can cause gastrointestinal problems and often is misdiagnosed by gastroenterologists, as had happened to me just months before, in April. It can bring your house down with pain, excruciating pain that is ever present during the most normal functions of everyday life. It is very dangerous to the physical, mental, and emotional well-being of a patient as well as the general well-being of her whole family. I had gotten my period twenty-three years earlier, a present from puberty that seemed like a bad joke that September morning. Now, decades later, on this evening, I sat in Dr. Seckin's office, hearing for the very first time that I had a disease called endometriosis, which could threaten my fertility. I had just turned thirty-six.

For twenty years, this powerful tissue had amassed and twined inside me, growing outward from my uterus, spreading through my body and coiling around my insides. It felt like it had choked and mutilated every part of my being. I wasn't crazy, or dramatic, and I didn't have a low threshold for pain. In fact, I probably had a high threshold for pain, and that may have been part of the problem. Dr. Seckin didn't understand why I wasn't writhing in pain outside his office. "I believe you when you say you think you have answered my questions honestly and sincerely," he pronounced very deliberately in his strong Turkish accent. "But what I see of your anatomy and the picture you are painting of your life seem very different."

So much was suddenly so clear. Just months before, in April, on our second wedding anniversary, I'd had to be rushed to the hospital late at night—the tissue had wrapped itself like a tourniquet around my small intestines, though I hadn't known then what was really happening. I had been in pain all day but didn't want to disappoint Salman, who had reserved a table at Bouley weeks before. To his credit, he suggested we stay home, but I wanted to celebrate with him. We both needed a good time together. I knew, too, that he expected to make love, something I wasn't sure I was capable of. Until recently, we had always been hungry for each other and could never get enough. Lately though, we had been fighting more and more about our lack of intimacy. I figured that after the meal and a bottle of red, he might tire out or, better yet, I might feel better. My plan was not very well thought out. The chef insisted on our having the tasting menu. A third of the way through, I asked the maître d' for a pillow. My lower back was throbbing and the pain was wrapping around to my abdomen, which was cramping, too. I thought the pillow might give me some support, or that I could find a more comfortable position leaning against it. With each course the waiter brought, my pain increased. I barely made it through the meal.

When we got home, I climbed up the stairs to the fourth floor. Halfway up, I began to have trouble breathing and stumbled. I made it to our bedroom, tore off my red jersey dress, and reached for the heating pad, which was always plugged in and waiting under my pillow. I turned on my side and doubled over. My husband came in and I told him that in addition to the back pain, I had begun cramping and that it really hurt. And I didn't know why. "Of course," he said. "How convenient for you. It's not your period and it's not ovulation. What is it this time?"

This didn't sound quite as cruel at the time as it seems now on the page. For years I had tried hard to hide my pain from others, even from him, and to dull my symptoms through denial and keeping busy. My mother told me from a very early age what her mother had told her: that this was just our lot in life. She said that the only thing to do was to try very hard not to let it affect any more of my life than it had to. So I compartmentalized the pain, tried to mostly sequester myself in bed until it subsided enough that I could get up. Now I understand that we were both feeling the effects of this vexing disease. To this day, my mother hasn't been officially diagnosed, but she has suffered the same mysterious pain, the same stab-in-the-dark surgeries. One doctor, ignorant of the cause of her suffering, threw up his hands and removed her appendix.

My husband never truly grasped the extent of my pain, in part because I took it for granted. Now Dr. Seckin was telling me that I probably had pain during sex. I wasn't sure that this was true. For the first several years together, our intimacy was fully gratifying. I don't ever remember having pain during sex. But I'd gotten so used to all the other pain that I didn't even identify it as pain anymore.

Recently I could remember my husband complaining that I rarely wanted to make love, and when I did it was only after we had been drinking. He felt justifiably rejected. I asked Dr. Seckin to call my husband and explain the disease's particulars, which I was only just beginning to understand. Coming from a doctor, I thought, the information would be less charged, more empirical. Then my husband would have to understand that I wasn't just making excuses. Yet my need for reinforcements, though I didn't understand it at the time, reflected a rift in our relationship that grew ever wider.

Now, after just two years of marriage and seven living together, our intimacy was fraught. I began to feel lonely, isolated by my pain. I started to feel happier—or more appropriately, less unhappy—when he wasn't around. In his presence, I felt as though I was not measuring up and was letting him down if I didn't do what or go where he wanted. By myself I was free to wonder what was increasingly wrong with my body without being made to feel like I was exaggerating. I was free to wallow in my malaise, and nurse myself without seeing the disappointment in his face. I needed to deal fully with what was happening to me. And I could only do that when I was alone.

That night of our second anniversary in April, he must have thought the pain I reported was in fact equivalent to my saying, "I don't feel like it and have to get up early." After a heated exchange of many words and much door slamming, he went to sleep in the room across the hall. Around midnight, I called an ambulance and Salman accompanied me to Mount Sinai hospital, where a gastroenterologist was waiting. Remember, this was *before* Seckin's diagnosis. The doctors were still clueless. The doctor who operated that night was like a landscaper, snipping off a small, unsightly root—"just scar tissue, perhaps from your earlier surgery for ovarian cysts, but you should be fine now," he said—while a massive, gnarled system still lurked beneath my house, threatening to crack the foundation. Sure enough, in the weeks and months after this surgery, the pain resumed. And my husband became increasingly frustrated with me. And I became more and more worried. Not only for my marriage, but also for my own body's health.

Now, just six months later, Dr. Seckin was telling me I wasn't crazy for not feeling like being intimate. He said every fiber of my being would be repelled by the idea of intimacy because of what was going on in my reproductive system and with my hormones. In fact, "I'm surprised you walked into my office on two feet," he said. I started to cry. I remember worrying, for a second, about ruining my makeup.

In the car inching its way down Fifth Avenue, toward Bergdorf Goodman and this glamorous party, I looked back on my past with a new understanding. This sickness, the "endo-whatever," had stained so much—my sense of self, my womanhood, my marriage, my ability to be present. I had effectively missed one week of each month every year of my life since I was thirteen, because of the chronic pain and hormonal fluctuations I suffered during my period. I had lain in bed, with heating pads and hot-water bottles, using acupuncture, drinking teas, taking various pain medications and suffering the collateral effects of them. I thought of all the many tests I missed in various classes throughout my education, the school dances, the jobs I knew I couldn't take as a model, because of the bleeding and bloating as well as the pain (especially the bathing suit and lingerie shoots, which paid the most). How many family occasions was I absent from? How many second or third dates did I not go on? How many times had I not been able to be there for others or for myself? How many of my reactions to stress or emotional strife had been colored through the lens of chronic pain? My sense of self was defined by this handicap. The impediment of expected pain would shackle my days and any plans I made.

I did not see my own womanhood as something positive or to be celebrated, but as a curse that I had to constantly make room for and muddle through. Like the scar on my arm, my reproductive system was a liability. The disease, developing part and parcel with my womanhood starting at puberty with my menses, affected my own self-esteem and the way I felt about my body. No one likes to get her period, but when your femininity carries with it such pain and consistent physical and emotional strife, it's hard not to feel that your body is betraying you. The very relationship you have with yourself and your person is tainted by these ever-present problems. I now finally knew my struggles were due to this condition. I wasn't high-strung or fickle and I wasn't overreacting.

All my life, I had had the sense that something was wrong and couldn't put my finger on it. I had seen college roommates pop two ibuprofen pills and skip off to basketball practice with no problems when they had their periods. I always wondered what was wrong with *me:* Why did I have such trouble dealing with one of the most basic and common functions Mother Nature handed all women? I heard my mother's voice echo in my head: "Because I had it, and your grandmother had it. It's just what happens."

In my mother's generation they would just take out all your plumbing if it got really bad. But now, "We can treat it with laparoscopic surgery, excise this problematic tissue and expel it from the body," said Seckin. "I am surprised you slipped through the cracks without any treatment this long."

If he was surprised, I was flabbergasted. I had dutifully gone to my gynecological checkups and not one doctor had ever brought up this disease. I even had two ovarian cysts removed at Cedars-Sinai Medical Center, where my Beverly Hills gynecologist had said that one of my cysts was "endometriotic," or blood-filled. But he never said the words "You have endometriosis. It is a condition that needs to be treated and monitored. It is a serious condition that can and will not only endanger your health and the proper function of your internal organs, but will also affect your fertility." In fact, endometriosis is one of the three major causes of infertility in women, and 10 percent of all women worldwide suffer from it.

As I reached the dinner, I tried to stuff back down all the emotions that had bubbled up, just as I'd stuffed away from view the pain and discomfort for all these many years. Just like I struggled to fit all my cosmetics back into my small evening bag after I dabbed and patched my face back together. The car door opened; a flashbulb went off. I hopped out of the car and fixed a smile on my face. At dinner, there were toasts and cheers as we looked out over Central Park, the first of the blue night's stars visible above the bony trees and the fallen autumn leaves.

Three weeks later, on the Wednesday before Thanksgiving, Dr. Seckin performed his first surgery. I picked the day in the hope I could recuperate over the long weekend without anyone knowing I'd been out of commission. At first, he guessed the surgery would take an hour and a half, and I'd be home the next morning and back at my desk by Monday.

I awoke to the sound of my own voice. I smelled the faint odor of mustard seeds and ginger. In the darkness of the hospital room, my mother, two aunts, an uncle, and various cousins kept vigil, leaning or sitting on every surface and quietly nibbling food from round tin containers. *Top Chef* was on the TV. There was a Thanksgiving marathon. Dr. Seckin came to speak to me in the recovery room after the surgery was over. In my anesthetized haze, I heard him say that my right fallopian tube had been rendered functionless from the buildup of endometriosis tissue. He asked if I knew that part of my left ovary had been removed during a previous operation. Incredibly, I didn't. I learned the surgery had taken four and a half hours, my kidneys were in stents, I had stitches on four major organs, and that of the nineteen biopsies performed, seventeen came back positive as deeply infiltrating endometriosis tissue (also known as DIE). Rather than an overnight stay, I spent five days in the hospital. Twenty-four hours after my discharge, my husband had to leave for a trip. "The show must go on, after all," he said.

My aunt Neela, who had flown in from India, and my mother, who had come from Los Angeles, cared for me, something they had done at different times throughout my life. Over the next two and a half months, as I lay bedridden on the top floor of our brownstone, they took turns, flying in and out. As they tended to me, my husband toiled in his office below. Over those many weeks, on my back staring at a white ceiling, I had ample time to think. There was nothing to distract me, no work I could do or ways to keep busy. Now, the thoughts that had exploded like little bombs in my head as I drove down Fifth Avenue that inky fall evening could no longer be muffled.

All those hours and days and weeks staring at that ceiling, looking back, revealed a new perspective on my years with Salman. Early on, we were so full of passion. Even when we fought, which we did quite a lot over matters both large and very small, I took it as evidence of the intensity of our love. He would slam doors and storm out, snatching a pillow from our bed and dramatically decamping to another room. *He's said his piece,* I'd think. *He'll cool off by morning.* Then I'd hear his fast footsteps on our creaky wood floor and he'd charge back in, like a rhinoceros up on its hind legs. I found these heated exchanges challenging and difficult. I had heard enough bad-tempered yelling from my stepdad in high school to last me a lifetime. I no longer wanted that as a part of my life. Nor did it help that my husband argued with the same lethal eloquence he had used to woo me. Of course, just because a point is well made, doesn't mean it's right. I was articulate enough but couldn't compete rhetorically. After a while, I was simply defiant.

Passion can come from many places, including but not limited to love. I don't doubt he loved me. Nor do I doubt that what seemed like a desire for me was also in part a desire for what I provided—an adoring audience.

Few people could resist his charm, the way he dominated a dinner party and made you glad you were there to listen. This made him a glorious friend and party companion. But after a party, everyone goes home. Me, I went home with him. I was the full-time, live-in audience.

As is the case with many creative people, his ego needed frequent tending. He is, without a doubt, a brilliant man and a great artist, yet somehow he lacked self-awareness and, tellingly, a sense of humor about himself. Every October, when the Nobel Prize winners were announced, he became moody and irritable. He was certain he was *nobélisable,* and every year I'd comfort him, cooing, "Of course you deserve it" and "Oh, they don't know what they're doing." I did feel he deserved it and the disappointment understandably cut him deeply. But then he'd say, "Yes, many great artists never get the Nobel," continuing on to list, without irony, those writers: "Proust, Joyce . . ."

My attention was proof of my devotion and my devotion was a balm for his insecurities. At first, I was grateful to be the object of such intense desire. Yet what's flattering in the first year can be suffocating in the eighth. I thought marriage might prove to him that I wasn't going anywhere.

To be fair, my husband didn't change during the eight years we were together. I knew what I was getting into. I think, however, that I changed, as do most women between twenty-eight and thirty-six. And because I'd been a model, enjoying six or so years of surreal, carefree existence, my twenties had been a sort of extended adolescence. When we met, he was already the man he'd always be. At twenty-eight, I was still becoming myself. Perhaps I didn't voice my unhappiness soon enough; rather, I spent more time feeling like a disappointment and scrambling to patch our cracks than I did considering whether he required an unreasonable level of tending. The tension grew worse as my work prospects grew brighter and I became, I guess, less portable. No longer could I be on his arm at every dinner and tribute. I had a second cookbook coming out, was hosting *Top Chef,* and had addressed the UN in support of the organization then called UNIFEM that advocated for women. Those achievements were my own. And I was proud of them.

All that time in bed and the locus of my sickness brought another matter into focus. I had never really decided whether I wanted children. Early on, Salman told me he didn't want to have another child. After all, he had two already. This made me wonder whether our relationship had legs. Ultimately, though, he relented. For me, he'd be open to it, and so I felt comfortable agreeing when one day we rolled out of bed after almost five years together and he wondered aloud, "Maybe we should get married."

"Are you asking me to marry you?" I asked.

"Yes, will you marry me?" he said.

Our honeymoon included a red carpet event in Cannes (my first) to help out his son Zafar, who was doing PR there, and a stop in Barcelona so he could give a speech. I was immune then to what this rather unromantic detour portended. And I didn't mind so much. I'd have said so if I did. What mattered was that we were together. As we walked the carpet, I watched the mass of photographers falling over one another as flashes flashed and shutters clicked with a constancy that produced a sound like an infestation of some strange insect trying to attract mates. I was no naïf at the time, no stranger to the spotlight or the paparazzi. I had paraded down the runaway in a bikini. I had cohosted a live TV show. Yet for some reason now, with cameras going off like automatic weapons, my worried thoughts—*why are they taking so many photos, like nature photographers trying to catch a hummingbird in flight, when we're standing still?*—became a physical presence. I couldn't breathe. Salman sensed something was wrong and I found comfort in his hand steady around my waist. For the next few years, until we divorced, I had panic attacks on the red carpet. In these moments I was captured being what I most feared I would become: an ornament or medal. I was not a model, host, actress, or advocate. I was wearing a sparkly dress and standing beside a great writer. I was worried, whether I knew it then or not, that without him I would simply disappear.

My laissez-faire attitude about motherhood began to change. The surgery brought a sense of urgency to my decision. If I did want kids, I would have to find out right away whether my body would even oblige. I'd also have to be sure I wanted to bring a child into this marriage. My husband was fifty-nine then. Aside from the logistical complexities of our relationship—he traveled often; his children lived in London; with which family would he spend holidays if I couldn't travel, as had been the case while I was bedridden?—there was my unhappiness. I was a child of divorce (two times over). I dreaded my child having the same experience. Before the operation, we had somehow managed to piece and patch together the relationship with the putty of our love. But now, I could no longer continue making those repairs. Even after the surgery and all of Dr. Seckin's talking to him, Salman didn't seem to grasp the disease's impact, on me or on our marriage. He was absent, emotionally and often physically. The women in my family shepherded me through recovery and made sure I was never alone.

I was left to grapple, however, with the most intimate effects, those that only a partner can know, by myself. I felt hollow, both in spirit and in body, my insides having been scalded, carved, and scraped out. I had been feeling guilty, like a bad wife, for not wanting to make love. It was this issue that was the nucleus of much of the strife between my husband and me. It must have been hard for him, after experiencing the intensity of my passion for him for all those years, to be confronted with my ebbing desire, my diminished wellness of being, and the increased distraction of my work.

But now the doctor had informed us that there was a tangible medical reason for my waning libido. It wasn't my fault. And it did not have anything to do with my love for him. Lying there bedridden, I felt that my sexuality was even more eroded than before the operation. I looked outside our window at the bare-limbed tree in the neighbor's backyard, stoic in northern light. I swam in an ocean of loneliness as I thought about my marriage and my future. I was drowning.

That loneliness then turned into anger. What about "in sickness and in health"? What about "I'm so sorry I gave you such grief when you were very ill"? What about "I'm sorry I didn't believe you on our anniversary, when the ambulance had to take you away"? Now, in retrospect, I can see how my husband suffered. The difference between two people who love each other as romantic partners and every other loving relationship is the sexual aspect of that union. At that time, I had just received the information that my fertility was in peril, I had been feeling like I had let down my husband for over a year (my body had failed me, but it had also failed him), and we were arguing almost every time I chose to pursue my own work instead of accompany him for his.

When I was finally well enough to leave the house, I went to see a divorce lawyer. It was not an easy trip, and not just because of the pain biting at my belly. To seek a divorce was to admit failure. It was to accept that the doubts my friends and family expressed early on—he had already been married three times; how would a relationship between two people of such unequal stature in age and accomplishment be equal or work out—were warranted. It was to confront the possibility that when we parted ways, I might disappear back into the relative obscurity from which I came. It was to tear my life in two, to leave the side of the man I had loved the most. Yet as always, my mother's story and will gave me hope. My mother, Vijaya (her name means "victory" in Sanskrit), had survived much worse. When my husband returned from his Christmas holiday in London, in January 2007, only to jet off again a few days later to the Jaipur Literature Festival,

I told him I wanted a temporary separation. "Well," he said, "you can have one, but it won't be temporary." I told him I had seen a lawyer, and he replied, "Then there's nothing to discuss."

By that April, I had recovered from my surgery, finished my cookbook, and flown to Miami to film the third season of *Top Chef*. Salman and I had reconciled a month back, provisionally. I thought then that ours was the greatest love story of my life and I couldn't bear to end it. We had agreed to work on our relationship. Three weeks into filming, my husband would fly down to celebrate our third wedding anniversary. I looked forward to it. But first I had work to do.

We had just finished a segment when I got word he had arrived and was waiting for me in the control room. "Thanks," I said. "Can you tell him I'm not done working, so I can just have a quick cigarette?" I forgot I was still wearing my mic. Salman could clearly hear me on the monitors. I had quit smoking when we first moved in together. I'd failed many times before. But he suffered from asthma and somehow it was easier to stop smoking for his health rather than for my own. As our marriage had started its painful undoing, I had resumed the insidious habit, keeping it a secret from him. I didn't want to add my smoking to the growing list of ways I disappointed him. After a long day of shooting and in the midst of another painful period, I needed a minute to myself, and some noxious relief.

I had both revealed my relapse and embarrassed him in front of my colleagues after he'd flown in from New York especially to see me. That night, when work wrapped, we fought. The row was exactly the same as the one we'd had a year earlier, after our anniversary dinner at Bouley, and just hours before I'd been carted away by an ambulance. It was the same one we'd had so many times before, the same one that had once caused him to lash out, calling me "a bad investment" during another fight in London on New Year's Eve in front of a friend. He wanted what I couldn't give him. I didn't feel like being intimate, and his constant irascibility because of that fact made me want to be even less so. This time, my empathy had waned, my guilty feelings about not performing my wifely duty outmatched by outrage. After all I'd been through medically. After all he'd seen. Nothing had changed. I fought feelings of failure, as a woman and as a wife. Still, I knew right then I had to leave.

I wasn't sure how we'd make the split public—an odd decision we had to consider. I was prepared to say that we parted amicably. He never gave me the privilege of deciding. "Salman Rushdie has agreed to divorce his wife, Padma Lakshmi, because of her desire to end their marriage," read the statement released by his literary agent. How businesslike. I was still in bed recovering from a subsequent endometriosis procedure at the end of June when a friend who had read the paper called to make sure I was okay. I had no idea any announcement had even been made. And so I was left with a mantra, a sort of haiku version of our relationship: I don't regret one day I spent with him, nor did I leave a moment too soon.

chapter 3

I'd moved into the Sorry Hotel over July Fourth weekend, while Salman was in London to visit his son Milan. I wanted to get out before they returned to New York. Sweet, little Milan, what would he think? Just a few years back I had taught him to roller-skate from our stoop so he could savor the city as I had when I was younger. I hated the thought of his breathing in the toxic atmosphere of loss and anger that then existed between Salman and me in our home. I wanted to talk to my stepson, to tell his that I still loved him, and that my leaving his father was not intended as a rejection of him; that I would still be there, if and whenever he wanted me, if his parents allowed it. I didn't get the chance. When I asked if I could speak to him, I was told by Salman that when he informed Milan, "She is leaving us," Milan had said, "Then I don't want to see her." *Us?* Who could blame a boy for siding with his father?

Days before I left, Dr. Seckin had performed yet another surgery, this one to excise the remaining endometrial tissue that he wasn't able to remove during the first. I was gaunt. A cocktail of sadness and medication made me nauseous and sapped my appetite. The stale smell of picked-at sandwiches and barely touched haystacks of French fries lingering on room service trays didn't help. I had been at the hotel for over a month by this time. Gavin Kaysen, the chef at Café Boulud, had been instructed by Daniel Boulud to look after me, and they often sent up trays filled with every single dessert on the menu. It was a gallant and kind gesture but did not restore my appetite.

I knew the trick to eating well was to cook for myself, and to that end I had selected this hotel room for its kitchenette. But I couldn't bear to turn on the stove. As thin as I was, I felt heavy and sluggish. I was paralyzed by sadness and self-doubt. Had I made a mistake getting married in the first place? Or had I given up too quickly? I had left a familiar unhappiness for a new, uncertain sort. I winced as I recalled my failings as a wife and I imagined confronting the people whose smiling faces populated our wedding photos. I tried to envision a future without the companion with whom I had spent half of my adulthood, my hope for a happy life eroding with each memory of my beloved.

Back on the floor, staring at those spilled kumquats scattered on the carpeting among the detritus of my life, I felt so inconceivably far from the days of intercontinental phone calls that reached into the night. I had left because I couldn't stay. There had been no shortage of love, no infidelity. It was a simple lack of empathy on both our parts. Racked by our own wounds and emotional fatigue, we could not soothe each other. And down we went, spiraling apart. I felt totally lost, out to sea, waiting for my thirty-seventh birthday, childless and now alone.

I had to do something to cut through the grayness around me, and the grayness inside. I picked up one of the kumquats and pressed my nail into its rind, releasing an aroma so faint I thought I'd imagined it. As a girl in Los Angeles, I made a game of stomping and squishing fallen kumquats as I walked to school. The kids on our block used to dare one another to eat them whole, plucked off the tree. Once in a while, one of us would take the dare, chomping down on the whole fruit, the sweet rind giving way to an explosion of bracingly sour pulp and the bitterness of broken seeds. Now, here in the hotel room, I licked the citric juice as it stung a torn cuticle. I could taste the sunshine and dirt of my mother's garden. I ached to be in her arms now, to bury myself in the cocoa-butter creaminess of her soft breasts. Whenever I despaired, I thought of my mother and my grandmother, both of whom had had lives much harder than mine.

My mother, Vijaya, was thirteen when her mother died. She spent the next six years shuttling among family members until she went to college. There she had a boyfriend, whose hand she would hold in secret when they thought no one was looking. But marriage for her, as it was for so many girls in that era, was to be arranged. Her father put an ad in the newspaper that joined countless other pithy summaries, just as they fill websites and the pages of *The Times of India* today. These were essentially matrimonial classifieds, with all the efficiency of a Craigslist posting for an old bookcase. My mom's went something like: "Groom wanted. Fair, lovely, college-educated (BSC), 25, 5'4", Tamil Brahmin Iyer girl seeks alliance with boy of similar and suitable background," plus her horoscope. Grooms to be were advertised with the same specs: complexion, education, age, height, background, caste, and sect. Desperation occasionally shone through these mundane details. In that era, if you spotted the phrase "caste no bar" (essentially meaning that any caste would do), then you knew the prospective bride or groom had baggage. A widow with children, say, couldn't limit herself to the higher castes.

A number of men showed up at the casting calls my grandparents held to inspect possible choices from ads that looked promising. My mother favored a tall, fair, handsome man who showed no fear in the face of her father. Quite the contrary: his cavalier manner included announcing that he belonged to an exclusive private club and peppering the conversation with a smattering of English swearwords she had never heard spoken aloud. To my grandfather, this man was insolent. To my mother, he was a rebel, the swaggering opposite of her secret college boyfriend who was too scared to hold her hand in public. Needless to say, my grandfather did not approve. She won the fight, but my grandfather was right in the end. A year later, they were married and on the day of the wedding, she saw him in the bathroom with his female cousin. At the time, she did nothing. *Once we're married and fall in love,* she thought, *he'll forget about her.* My mother was a nurse, well versed in the bodily aspects of the birds and the bees, but naïve about love.

Less than a year later, when she found out she was pregnant, her husband dragged her to the doctor, who refused to perform an abortion on a woman so clearly there under duress. I wince now when I think about how I almost wasn't. Twenty-five years later, when I first met my biological father, I asked him to explain himself. He regretted it, he said, but at the time he didn't want to bring a child into such a troubled marriage. Only after my own marriage revealed itself to be doomed did I understand his inclination, if not his actions.

During my mother's pregnancy, they moved into an apartment just a couple of floors above the kissing cousin. He'd often leave my mother home alone, slinking in many hours after work ended and lying about where he'd been. One night, his friend Krishnan dropped by while he was out. Disturbed by the sight of a very pregnant woman left home alone, Krishnan stayed with her for hours. He was gone when my father finally stumbled home. She confronted him. "Where have you been?" she asked. "I told you, I was with Krishnan," he said.

I was born in Safdarjung Hospital in New Delhi. My mother endured thirty-six excruciating hours of labor unmitigated by an epidural. She gave birth in a hospital bed, not at home as my grandmother had, but otherwise it was as natural as could be. I learned of her long labor from an aunt only a few years ago. Throughout our many rows, my mother never wielded it as a rhetorical weapon. All she ever said was, "Once I saw you, *kanna,* it didn't hurt at all."

My parents were fighting constantly by the time I turned one. My grandfather came to the house to help resolve their disputes. Divorce was anathema to conservative Indian culture then. It barely existed in the cultural vocabulary, religious or otherwise. Most couples stuck out marriage, through thick and thin, infidelity and abuse. Yet when he heard my father spit, "Your daughter is ready to lick my boots," my grandfather sided with his daughter over tradition and took her and me back to Delhi. They divorced a year after. But because divorce was so unheard of in middle-class Indian society, people looked at divorcées with a sort of incredulous shock and wonder, as if they were somehow criminals. They were ostracized from everyday life because of an invisible scarlet D hovering over them.

Meanwhile, Second Wave feminism in the United States was changing attitudes about how women were treated in the workplace and in society, and how unmarried women were perceived in particular. Women were challenging age-old notions of their place in the world. Western media was full of unafraid, smart American women who published magazines, were marching in DC, and were generally making a lot of noise. No such phenomenon had reached our Indian shores. I'm sure my mother had read about the ERA movement, *Roe v. Wade,* and bra burnings. She, too, wanted the freedom to earn a living in a country where she wouldn't be a pariah because of her marital status. We could have a fighting chance at surviving independently in the United States, versus being dependent on her father or a future husband in India. Conservative as he was, my grandfather K. C. Krishnamurti, or "Tha-Tha," as I called him in Tamil, had encouraged her to leave my father after he witnessed how she had been treated. He respected women and loved his daughter and it must have broken his heart to see the situation she had married into. He, too, wanted us to have a second chance at happiness. America, devoid of an obvious caste system and outright misogyny, seemed to value hard work and the use of one's mind; even a woman could succeed there. My grandfather was a closet feminist.

So, when I was two, my mother left India for America. She couldn't afford to bring me with her. She couldn't care for a young daughter while she studied for her local nursing license and worked in a hospital. She would spend the next two years diligently working in quiet agony, preparing a life for me. Tha-Tha and his second wife, my grandmother Rajima, raised me back home. While my mother prepared a life for us in New York, my grandfather tutored me for that life back in New Delhi. For those two years, I would effectively see neither of my parents.

My grandmother tells me that long after the other kids had stopped playing and gone inside, I'd sit by the fence that enclosed our building's courtyard in New Delhi. She would call me in and I'd shake my head. When asked what I was waiting for, I'd say, "I'm waiting for my mom to come home from office in America," pronouncing the last word "Ahm-ree'-KAI." In Tamil, my native language, you add the suffix "*kai*" to a plant to refer to its vegetable. I didn't know America from bitter gourd. I certainly didn't know it was a place across an ocean. I waited with my grandparents while my mother worked to make a better life for us. She sent for me when I was four.

I finally rejoined my mother on Halloween night in 1974, exactly two years to the day after she herself had first deplaned at JFK. She picked me up at the airport wearing a poncho that she'd knitted. She had a blanket draped over her arm, because she feared I would suffer in the New York cold.

On the way home in a cab, we passed many children in costume—witches and clowns and Batmen. I thought they were beggars, like the urchins on the streets in Delhi who would dress up and perform for rupees. But there were so many! We reached my mother's apartment, at 405 East Eighty-Third Street in Manhattan. Inside near the door I noticed a bowl of candy, which I assumed was for me. But the doorbell kept ringing and my mother kept handing over *my* candy to these costumed kids! I was horrified until she explained the holiday. *Ahm-ree'-KAI,* I thought, *a magical place where kids get candy just for dressing up!*

She gave me a very short tour of her one-bedroom apartment, which was much smaller than my grandparents' home in Delhi. Of course, that didn't matter to me. My mother's presence more than made up for the lack of space. We lay together in her queen-size bed, under brightly colored covers, and I fell asleep excited—about candy and clowns, about our new life together. She had sculpted the mist, the way those who have no choice do. She had willed a life for the two of us in a new land.

My new life brought many changes—a new city, and my mother's new boyfriend—but none as jarring as suddenly being deposited in the land of omnivores. My family members, Brahmins all of them, were strict vegetarians. In India, a large vegetarian population meant loads of options at the restaurants and street stalls. When I arrived in the States, I wouldn't even consider eating meat, despite my mother's pleading. It was the seventies and meat was considered healthy. She also wanted her daughter to explore and enjoy the city and its food along with her. The food at these restaurants was either too meaty or too strange for me at the time, and early on it was a struggle to feed me. Of course, she and her boyfriend, a Punjabi cab driver from Queens, couldn't afford to go out *and* pay for a sitter, so I went out with them, too. (Dragging a kid along, even well past her bedtime on a weeknight, is squarely within seventies Indian tradition, which claims, disingenuously or not, that routine is not nearly as important as familial togetherness.)

My mom did make sure that her culinary wanderlust took us exclusively to restaurants that had rice, virtually the only thing I'd eat. And so I became New York's most practiced rice aficionado. At Mañana's on First Avenue, my mom ate tacos as I focused on a heap of red-hued grains and beans. At the Japanese place near the Russian Tea Room, where customers sipped soups from small bowls cupped in their hands, I ate rice doused with soy sauce and Tabasco. I liked sitting on the floor and watching all the men struggle to remove their chunky-heeled boots and sit comfortably with their dates.

In India, we always sat on the floor at home and took off our shoes before entering the house, so I was perfectly at ease there. At a long-gone Armenian place in the East Forties, I ate pilaf and cucumbers. And whatever I ate, I shoveled into my mouth with my right hand, just as I'd learned to do in India. Except for the occasional flat wood spoon that came with ice cream cups, I had never really used or even been presented with silverware before I got to America. Spoons and forks took me a while to get the hang of.

We soon found our groove, though. Namely, we discovered that uniquely American phenomenon: the Salad Bar. Not only was there a seemingly infinite amount of food, not only was it all food I could eat—canned beets, kidney and garbanzo beans, onions and chutneys ("dressings," my mom corrected me)—but you could also eat as much of it as you wanted. I'd pile my plate high, with as many colors of foods as I could, and then go back for more.

In India, a meal was not a meal unless there was rice. In America, a meal seemed not to be a meal unless there was bread. Americans, it seemed to me, ate a lot of sandwiches. I was four when I made my first sandwich. I was hungry and hunger makes you get creative. What I really wanted was a cheese and chutney sandwich, an Indian classic that the British pervert with cheddar and super-sweet mango relish. So I rummaged through my mom's fridge and found a foil-wrapped block of Philadelphia cream cheese. I spread it on bread and added a good squirt of ketchup. One of my favorite vegetarian discoveries, falafel, always came tucked into bread, like a sandwich in the shape of a little purse. Since it was a sandwich, I assumed falafel was an American food, despite the belly-dancing music blaring from the joints that sold it. Most sandwiches, though, I thought of as "pink in bread." The pink was either dark (hot dog) or light (bologna). I remained a lotus-eater until well into puberty, but when I did succumb to my mother's cajoling as well as to some good, old-fashioned American peer pressure, my training wheels were made of bologna. The Formica of meat, bologna is meat denatured—no bones, no flesh, no blood. It doesn't resemble anything mortal, which helped it go down, as did lots of mustard. But even before I gave up the ghost, my mom and I would frequent hot dog vendors, the *chaatwallahs* of New York City. As we named topping after topping—mustard and kraut and ketchup and relish—vendors would ask yet again, "So you want it *without* the hot dog?" *Yes,* we'd shake our heads in unison.

Not long after I arrived, my mother married her cabbie boyfriend, V., at City Hall. I was their only guest. After they married, we moved to Elmhurst, Queens—East Elmhurst Avenue, to be precise. I remember almost every address, to the letter, at which I've lived. Perhaps I need to remember as a way of keeping track of where I have come from, since I shifted a lot between the U.S. and India. I pass the place every time I go to JFK Airport. My apartment in SoHo today is merely a few miles away from these graffitied buildings, but the forty-year journey between the two feels as long as the distance between the earth and the moon.

Our building faced another identical building and the apartments in both were filled with immigrants. I'd explore the halls on my own, chatting up the old ladies shuffling around the courtyard. "Who do you live with?" I'd wonder aloud, and the widow would say, "Sweetie, I live alone." No daughter to soak your feet in hot water after work (a concept I borrowed from the sitcom *Alice*)? No husband to take you out for kebabs? So I'd go back to our apartment, choose one of my mother's brightly colored scarves, and present it to the widow. I did this with many women. The next time one of these women saw my mother, she'd thank her with watery eyes for the beautiful scarf. "What scarf?" my mother would say.

The buildings teemed with children, a blessing for my mother. The winter would otherwise have had me cooped up in the apartment, yet I spent weekends roaming the buildings with a gang of Indian kids. We'd occasionally get a hold of some *chaat* and eat it in the halls—*chaat* is street food, and these were our streets. Shoveling it into our mouths with our hands, we'd earn funny looks from the non-Indian kids.

Some nights, I'd join my mom and V. at a Manhattan movie theater that showed Indian movies and, as a lucrative sideline, they would set up a folding table next to the concession stand, from which they sold samosas, homemade chutneys, and hot chai. I helped out, mainly by fanning the napkins (as V. taught me to do from his bartending days, using a glass on its side) and devouring their wares, though at that age, one samosa made a meal. I spent most of the time haunting the balcony seats.

I spent my days at Resurrection Ascension School in Elmhurst, Queens—which always struck me as an awfully long name for an elementary school, nearly impossible to get right at age five. My kindergarten teacher was Ms. Schliff, and my first class photo shows me wearing a lime-green, white, and black striped sweater, sporting a shag flip, and clasping Alistair Cooke's book *America*.

Every day after school, I went to our neighbor Elena's apartment for three hours, until my mom got off from work and picked me up. Because I refused to eat any of the meat-heavy options at school, I also walked to Elena's every day to have lunch. Elena got paid to babysit multiple kids in our building and had no shame about putting us to work. I got lucky. While some of the kids were assigned to pick lint from her maroon shag carpet, I got to help in the kitchen. Elena was Peruvian and she'd often enlist me to peel potatoes for empanadas. She let me mash the boiled potatoes with chopped parsley and adobo. I loved the smell of freshly chopped parsley, the satisfaction of crushing the vegetables, and the neat packaging of it all in pastry. The result would remind me of samosas and *aloo tikkis*.

For lunch, I subsisted on cans of Campbell's condensed soup, which my mother would lug to Elena's by the bagful. Very few Campbell's soups were vegetarian, so my options were limited to cream of mushroom, cream of potato, and the vegetarian version of alphabet soup, which made up for its lack of creaminess with its seductive letter-shaped noodles. I had tried cream of celery but winced at its metallic taste, and cream of cheddar was as gruesome as it sounds. I was disappointed to learn that the intriguingly titled "Pepper Pot" soup contained beef stock.

Later, when I was a few years older, I started experimenting with the soups on my own. Whenever I was stuck at home and hungry, I could always pop open a can, mash the contents with milk or water, heat it all in a pot on the stove, and go to town. At first, my biggest challenge as a cook was successfully eradicating the lumps. Then, it was turning the soups into something worth eating. Along with the cream cheese and ketchup sandwich, one of my first creations as a cook was cream of potato doctored up with chopped jalapeño chilies. Soon I started adding dried herbs like oregano, mixing in a can of alphabet soup, and drizzling in the liquid from pickled jalapeños. I still save this spiced vinegar for brightening anything that needs it in my fridge today.

V., my mother's second husband, was a pretty darn handsome North Indian with fair skin and an occasional beard. A card-carrying member of the Playboy Club—a sophisticated quality at the time—he had a thing for chunky-heeled pleather boots, bell-bottoms, and wildly printed shirts open one button too many. He wore a chain with a medallion of the goddess Durga that nestled in the exposed tuft of hair on his chest.

He drove a yellow cab by day and went to radiology school at night. My mother helped him, bought him a car (she did not know how to drive at the time), and over several years used her green card status to sponsor his mother's, brother's, sister's, and brother-in-law's immigration to America. Many of them stayed with us, at various times. My mother worked days as a nurse at Sloan Kettering and studied for a master's degree at night, all the while helping to support a household of in-laws. Determined that I not lose touch with our family or culture, she somehow found money to fly me to India every summer without fail, and packed my suitcase full of gifts for all my relatives, including but not limited to bubble gum and chess timers, peanut butter and Pringles, vegetable peelers and can openers, bras and books, fashion magazines, LPs, sneakers and jeans, hair elastics and accessories, mascara, powder blush, perfume, eye shadow palettes, myriad of eye and lip pencils, and wool socks for my grandfather. She had an unmatched ability to cram consumer goods between my T-shirts and jeans.

Some mornings, when V. was up early to start a day of driving, he would take me to school. My friends at Resurrection Ascension must have thought I was posh because I arrived at school in a cab. One winter morning, he dropped me off so early that the school hadn't yet opened. It was snowing and I got so cold waiting in the schoolyard that I wandered into the adjoining church for shelter. The organ droned as parishioners attended morning mass. As a Hindu, I had never observed Mass, been baptized, or taken Communion. At school, while the other children rehearsed the choreography of confirmation services and taking Communion, the nuns made me sit in the last rows of pews. Yet that morning, the lone schoolkid among the early worshippers, I found an empty pew near the front and looked on as the priest spoke. I got up and sat down when others did, so as not to look disrespectful or like I didn't belong there. Suddenly, the worshippers waded toward the pulpit, and I was herded along with them. Then I was in front of the priest and he was smiling and placing something on my tongue.

I was used to eating as part of religious ceremonies. At home and in Hindu temples, our offerings, called *prasadam,* were fruits or sweets or spicy, savory snacks. What the priest fed me was the strangest *prasadam* I had ever had. Confused by the profound lack of flavor, I wondered whether I was meant to ingest this dusty object that possessed all the appeal of a piece of felt. I was suddenly afraid. Perhaps this was a decoy *prasadam.* Perhaps the priest knew I was an impostor, feigning piousness for shelter from the cold. Feeling guilty for being at church, where I knew I shouldn't be, I was scared to chew, so my mouth hung slightly open, heavy with the religious contraband. I returned to the pew and sank in my seat, trying to disappear, the stale disc melting to a gruesome mush on my tongue. I was discovered there, cowering, by a stern nun, my first-grade teacher. "What are you doing here?!" she said, quickly divining the answer and prying my mouth open with a bony finger. "Dear, you can't take Communion," she went on. "You are not Catholic!" I thought I might pee in terror, but just then, the sister burst out laughing. I believe this was the only time I ever saw her smile.

Our apartment in Queens was often packed with my mom's in-laws. Many nights I shared a bed in the second bedroom with a twenty-something relative of V.'s, a state of affairs that, to people like us who were used to living far too many to an apartment in India, seemed relatively normal. I was seven. One night I woke up to his hand in my underpants. He took my hand and placed it inside his briefs. I don't know how many times it had happened before, since I suspect I slept through some incidents. Even the incident I remember rather well remains blurred at the edges, a sort of half dream. I had shown signs of distress. There was a space between my headboard, the bed, and the wall where I'd occasionally toss pink pistachio shells. Once I peed in this space, defiling the place where I'd been defiled. My mother was shocked to see the mess of pink shells and urine that finally stank up the place. After I told her about the family member's abuse, she told her husband. One day, I arrived home after school and V. made me lie on the living room divan to demonstrate by pantomime what had happened. The next thing I knew, I was on a plane to Madras. This was shortly after I finished second grade.

Many potential explanations exist for my decampment. For one, my mother had been part of the team that had secretly treated the Shah of Iran at Sloan Kettering. For that, she received death threats, including a call to our apartment. "We know where you live with your daughter," a voice had hissed. At the time, however, all I knew was that I had opened my mouth and got sent away. My mother was right to immediately put distance between me and that man, of course. In retrospect, however, he should have been the one to go. Years later, in tears, my mother would acknowledge this grave mistake.

My grandmother Raji—or Rajima, as I called her, because she was still too young to be called *paati*—had led a life harder still than my mother's. Though *I* never knew any other grandmother, Rajima was not my mother's mother. My mother's mother died when she was thirteen and my grandfather married Raji three years later. One of sixteen children, in the deep-southern district of Tanjore, she was just another hungry mouth for her parents to feed. She was fourth in line but her mother became pregnant with another child soon after her birth in an effort to produce a male heir. A male child had been born but died before the age of two. Raji was not a boy, nor was she fair-skinned like her younger sister Vasantha, who would later receive dance training, an investment by her father made in the offspring most likely to provide some return. Her parents sent her away as a young girl to live with an aunt who had no children. Rajima was probably sent away to give her mother some breathing room, as caring for several kids while also being pregnant put a strain on her health. When she came back at five years old, she did not call her mother Amma. She did not know her; she could not bring herself to call her Mom.

Instead, she eventually acted as mother to her twelve younger siblings. A natural-born teacher, Raji honed her skills by shepherding her brothers and sisters through their studies. At age eighteen, she signed up for a Montessori teacher training course and later found a job as a teacher and even started a school in her province where there had never been one prior. The job became her ticket to independence. It staved off an arranged marriage, at least long enough for her to develop her career. It took her from Tanjore to Madras to New Delhi, the nation's capital in the north. By thirty years old she had, unlike many Indian women of her day, seen a bit of the world before duty called.

Raji had come home from teaching in New Delhi for summer vacation when a meeting was arranged by my grandfather's sister. She had heard that my grandmother's family was looking to marry off an older daughter. Raji's younger sister (the dancer) Vasantha's husband, a business magnate named V. D. Swamy, arranged it from the girl's side. My grandmother was doing well, but in those days an unwed woman pushing thirty was not looked well upon. My grandmother was earning money and helping her older sister Kamala, with whom she lived in Delhi. But a single woman always presented the potential danger of being an added dependent to her family. Back then, a woman was not seen as a full adult, but rather a ward either of her own family or of her in-laws. She would have been a constant liability until her future was settled with marriage. My widower grandfather went to see Raji in Tanjore with my young mother in tow one evening in early summer. They talked extensively that evening and the potential groom's party left the next day.

Then for some days, there was radio silence. My grandmother could not stand the suspense so she took matters into her own hands. She must have liked him in that first meeting, because she boldly wrote a letter to my grandfather. He was taking too long to decide. "If we don't get married I have to go back soon to Delhi to my job, or I will lose it," my grandma wrote. "So make up your mind either way." My grandfather, who was at that time touring the south for work, came back to Tanjore and visited my grandmother again without his daughter. He spoke to her father, went to the jeweler's that night for the *thali,* or ceremonial wedding necklace, and asked a local shopkeeper to open a store after hours so he could buy her a wedding sari. The very next morning they got hitched.

Love and passion begat marriage in my world. Yet in my grandparents' world, marriage began with practicality. My grandfather told me proudly of that day he first met my grandmother. He interviewed her, posing little riddles to test her common sense. "Supposing you have to take the children to school and you're late and it's supposed to rain," he said. "Would you take a taxi or a bus?" My grandmother said, "Well, first I'd take an umbrella." Ice cream in Central Park, this was not.

With quiet resolve and great political skill she navigated her new household, which was already populated by three children, two boys and the brooding teenager that was my mom at sixteen. Raji managed to feed them all as well as her own daughter, Neela, who came on the scene in 1963. She maintained her bright demeanor even when the number of mouths grew to ten, including grandchildren and daughters-in-law, by 1977, and when on weekday mornings four girls were still naked and late for the school bus and two men did not yet have their lunches packed.

After my grandfather retired from government service, he moved the family from New Delhi to Madras. I had always assumed my grandmother was happy to be down south again; years later I learned she actually preferred the north, with its milder climate and more modern ways. But as with so much of life, she had little choice. No one ever asked her what she wanted. She existed where life had taken her, and she chose to get on with it. From the start, my grandmother did not expect love, though she came to be loved deeply and respected by her husband. She returned his affection in her own ways, though she still slept best alone on the marble floor of the bedroom without a mattress or blanket. In fact, because of the heat, she relished getting all her work done and napping in the afternoon on the floor in her bedroom, alone. Neela and I occupied the space below their bed at night, so afternoons were the only time she had to herself.

Our family home did not ever have air-conditioning and the marble floor was the coolest place to sleep, especially in the pre-monsoon heat. When my husband and I got engaged, I brought him home to meet my folks in India. His upbringing in an upper-class Muslim family in Bombay had been much more privileged than what we were used to down south. I was afraid the heat would be too much for him. He was a sweater to boot. I had air-conditioning put in the other bedroom, with my grandfather complaining the whole way about the electric bills. Since then, during visits we've all congregated in the one room with air-conditioning, leaving my grandmother to enjoy, finally, the solace of her cool marble floor anytime she wants peace.

Raji did not expect happiness, though she could pluck from deep within the appreciation of simply being fed, clothed, sheltered, and regarded. I once asked her if she was happy. "That depends on what I am able to get done today," she said, laughing. She told me that the completion of her daily tasks was the only thing she felt she had control over. They were a form of meditation, of salve. Kept busy, she had no time to ruminate and no time for opinions, certainly not feminist ones. I pressed her: "I mean, are you happy *with your life*, Rajima?" "I don't know," she said uncomfortably, as if she'd never really considered such a question. "When there is little you can do, you do what you can." Happiness for my grandmother seemed to be a verb rather than a noun. She had so little control over her own life. Yet she took control, out of thin air for herself, when she could.

I thought of her counsel as I sat on the floor of my room in the Sorry Hotel. *Just do one thing,* I told myself, *complete one task.* I crawled through the cardboard labyrinth, collecting as many kumquats as I could in a floppy green hat I grabbed from a half-emptied box, gathering the brim around the fruit like a beggar's pouch. In the hotel room's kitchenette, I peered into the fridge, which I had stocked when I arrived but hadn't so much as opened for days. Rummaging through the produce drawer, I pulled out some green chilies, a knob of ginger, and a few bags of leaves and seeds from an Indian market. I knew one thing I could do. I had a deadline from *Gourmet* magazine hanging over me, which, in my stupor, I had willfully ignored. At the time I cursed myself for signing up to do a holiday-gifting story that entailed recipes for chutneys and pickles. But God bless the kitchen saint Ruth Reichl, the magazine's editor, for unwittingly helping to get me off my ass, and my mother for sending those kumquats.

If I could at least make a big batch of some sauce, some condiment, then it would do two kinds of work for me. I could meet my professional obligation, and I could use that sauce to bring *some* sunshine back into my life. I could lift myself, at least gastronomically, from the gray. I could turn that hatful of dusty citrus into something golden. And indeed, the kumquat chutney I ended up making is what woke me up in a sense. I'm certain that in large part, it had to do with the fact that my grandmother used to make a similar tangerine peel chutney I loved when growing up. I could use the fruits my mother gifted me, in my grandmother's recipe, as a potent anti-dote to my sense of being adrift, lost at sea, unmoored. I always thought that what Rajima did with those cast-off peels was a metaphor for how she dealt with her arranged marriage. She transformed those peels, with palm sugar for sweetness and tamarind for tang, into something precious.

When I was growing up, fresh fruit was expensive for us. My grand-mother was allowed to buy fruit only when my grandfather was feeling flush. During mango season, she would occasionally hand out pits after she'd carved the fruits and I'd suck those pits for half an hour, trying to get every last bit of flesh.

When we visited other people's homes we often took a small basket of bananas, apples, or pomegranates as gifts the way Westerners might bring a bottle of wine. My grandfather would occasionally spring for fruit when a religious ceremony, or *puja*, took place in our home. But in general, he thought fruit a frivolous luxury. In fact, even on religious holidays, when we needed a *prasadam,* or offering, he preferred a liquidy, sweet rice or noodle pudding called *payasam.* Fruit was expensive, but the milk and sugar for *payasam* could be purchased with our ration cards.

I often thought that Rajima's vociferous haggling with the poor spindly-legged fruit and vegetable vendor each morning was for my grandfather's benefit. Whatever the reason, she was good at it. By the time she finally bought a handful of small, sweet tangerines, she had weaseled her way into a free handful of green chilies and a knob of ginger. She always left with a few tangled branches of curry leaves, for which she never paid or haggled. That sweet fool gave them without fuss with every purchase, just for the pleasure of her daily verbal thrashing, as predictable as the noon heat and as welcome as a cold shower.

My grandmother cooked every meal fresh, not only because she believed it produced healthier and tastier food but also because she didn't grow up with the luxury of a fridge. In fact, she never had one until her thirties. Even after the fridge came, her routine didn't change. She didn't know any other way. Having so many mouths to feed meant she was almost always cooking. She made the chutney with cast-off peels along with whatever ginger, chilies, and curry leaves hadn't been used up for the evening meal. I yearned for this chutney far more than for the sweet fruit. While everyone else quietly ate their stir-fried curries and soupy lentils ladled over rice, I fixed my attention on a bowl of white rice mixed with sour homemade plain yogurt and a heap of that exquisite chutney. Rajima, or Jima as we often called her, turned a blind eye to my selfish hoarding of the chutney, because no one else moaned over it with sufficient ecstasy. My young palate was Jima's best audience.

Back in that hotel room, thirty years later, I made a big batch of kumquat chutney. To generate the recipe, I used a ton of freshly chopped ginger and hot green chilies and simplified the spices, mostly because I didn't have them all on hand. But it worked. I spooned a bit into my mouth, the fresh chilies and tart citrus jolting my palate free from stupor. Soon I found myself at the market again, buying pearly scallops, heaving fennel bulbs and sweet potatoes into my basket. I also bought goat cheese and butter, hoping to put some weight back on. I savored that first marigold-hued, glazy dollop, and thought of all the things I could do with this golden chutney.

What I did with those kumquats became a strategy I call upon whenever I want to eat well but can't for reasons of time, weakness, or inertia. As soon as I can conjure the energy, I make up a big batch of some flavorful sauce, a sort of "mother sauce," shall we say, and use it throughout the week by the tablespoon or cup to give life to simple food. The French have masterfully used sauces as the base to make their dishes for centuries. They have hundreds, many created—or consolidated, anyway—by the early-nineteenth-century chef Antonin Carême. Then those were whittled down by the great Auguste Escoffier into what we now know as the five mother sauces of French cuisine. It's funny to me that most of the cooking in the world is done by women, and yet when you look at modern Western cuisine, it's largely based on what a few dead Frenchmen have opined to be the correct way of doing things. It's funny how these old European men used a label like "mother sauce" when there were no women to be found anywhere near those old professional kitchens. Cooking was something women did to nourish and nurture their families, whereas for men it was largely something they did professionally to gain money and status. *My* version of a mother sauce actually comes from my foremothers, from the fruits of my mother's garden, and is based on a recipe handed down from my grandmother. I have always associated cooking with womanhood. At that moment, in August 2007, when I did not feel so womanly, with my insides carved out and my marriage a failure, the only thing I could take pleasure in was that golden sauce.

kumquat and ginger chutney

Serves 8 to 10

2½ pounds fresh kumquats, quartered and pitted
2 tablespoons kosher salt
½ cup canola oil
1 teaspoon fennel seeds
1 dozen fresh medium curry leaves, torn into small pieces
3 tablespoons minced fresh ginger
8 small green serrano chilies, chopped or sliced in half lengthwise
6 whole fresh kaffir lime leaves
½ teaspoon sambar or Madras curry powder (I prefer 777 brand)
½ cup water, plus more if needed
2 tablespoons light brown sugar

In a large bowl, mix the kumquats with the kosher salt. Let them rest for 2 to 3 hours, or overnight in the fridge, if possible.

Heat the oil in a deep pan for a few minutes on medium heat. Add the fennel seeds. When they sizzle and darken slightly, after about 2 to 3 minutes, add the curry leaves, ginger, and chilies, frying and stirring for just a minute or two. Then add the kaffir lime leaves and kumquats. Stir well. After 5 minutes add the curry powder and stir again.

After 5 minutes more, stir in the water and sugar.

Reduce the heat to medium-low and cook covered for 10 minutes, stirring intermittently to ensure the chutney does not stick to the bottom of the pan. If this happens, stir in more water, ¼ cup at a time, but the mixture should remain thick and gooey. Cook just until the chutney has a chunky jamlike consistency.

chapter 4

Maybe that old adage about not being able to have a good apartment, a good relationship, and a good job at the same time is true. I had been living at the Sorry Hotel for several months. I had no relationship, but I was thankful for my job on *Top Chef*. Indeed, because the show filmed in a different location every season, we basically moved to that town for those weeks and set up camp like gypsies. So this scenario was a blessing in disguise, because at least for those weeks my hotel expenses would be covered. I put most of my belongings in storage and went to Chicago for my third season. At the time, I wasn't making enough to live on from the show alone, but I was making ends meet (barely) by piecing together the writing, the book advance, and, believe it or not, still the occasional modeling gig. On bad days, which were many, I felt lost and displaced, like when I first moved back to the States from Italy at the end of my twenties—except scarier, because now I had just turned thirty-seven. On good days, which were few, I felt the same as when I was a young model in Europe just after college. I didn't know what the future held in store for me, but I felt hopeful. My second cookbook was being published and I had recently secured a two-year contract with Pantene.

Top Chef was really starting to take hold in popular culture. My job meant a whole new world was revealed to me—besides learning restaurant techniques and terminology, I had the opportunity to meet incredible chefs, like Daniel Boulud and Wylie Dufresne, and also to share meals with them. I got to talk shop all day long, to gush adjectives when describing a course of food the way tennis fans might describe a stunning serve, the way I used to coo over Dior and Yves Saint Laurent.

I ate my excitement. I was a puppy dog, wide-eyed and eager, so thrilled to be at the table that I overdid it. Here were these talented professional cooks vying to outdo one another, wielding racks of lamb and pork belly and cream—ingredients designed to make food as lush and rich and irresistible as possible. This was food I would never dream of making at home. I was, and still am, an enthusiastic home cook. Nothing special, just someone who hopes that guests will like my lentil recipes. These chefs cooked with liquid nitrogen, duck fat, and sous-vide. I got to eat it all beside our head judge, Tom Colicchio, and Eric Ripert, and knew I had a chance to learn from these culinary giants. I'd take a bite of sweetbreads or escolar and timidly express my ambivalence. Tom would dub it exceptional and ask me why I didn't like it. Eric would disagree with Tom, and they'd discuss the finer points of searing, poaching, and seasoning. And I was left eager to understand why they knew it was improperly cooked by what they were tasting, and why I didn't. I would taste the dish again as they playfought. And then again. That became a pattern with me: when in doubt, I took another bite.

While part of my overindulgence came from my lack of experience, the rest came from self-doubt. I've always been intent on proving that I wasn't just a five-foot-niner plucked at random from the catwalk. I had, or at least I thought I had, some credibility. I'd written two cookbooks and had hosted food documentaries and a cooking show on the Food Network. But still I worried. I had more than a touch of imposter syndrome. Tom had proven his chops cooking for great chefs and heading up more than a couple of restaurants that were well respected in New York. Gail had gone to culinary school and worked as an assistant to Daniel Boulud and to Jeffrey Steingarten before joining *Food & Wine* magazine. Our show was the sister show to *Project Runway,* and it made sense that a model hosted a show on fashion. But I didn't want people to think that Bravo had just put another model into the same format for their new food competition show.

I got looks at first from a few of the guest judges who didn't know me at all—most of them accomplished chefs—that virtually screamed, "Why the hell are *you* here?" I felt they thought I was nothing more than a pretty face. And ever since my first cookbook came out, I'd heard the tired complaint: What does a model know about eating? So as soon as the food came out, I ate like I had something to prove. I ate to the point of discomfort. Sure, I hadn't broken down a side of beef or cooked on the line. But I'd eaten and learned about good food all over the world—the finest *bastillas* in Marrakesh, tons of meals in Paris bistros, fresh pasta made by expert hands in Milan, the best *biryani* in Hyderabad, and the most exhilarating *chaat* in Delhi.

My love for food was born in India, where I spent the first four years of my life and many summers afterward. The vivid flavors I experienced there will forever be the standard to which I hold any food I eat today. Perhaps my most formative food experiences happened when my mother sent me back to Madras to study for the year. It was also during this time that my mother was divorced by my stepfather V., because he did not believe what she and I had told him about what happened to me in my bed.

When I arrived in Madras I immediately entered third grade (or "standard," as it's known there) at St. Michael's Academy, the new local Catholic school, in the middle of the school year. It was an English medium school but students were required to study a second Indian language from kindergarten on. I spoke Tamil more or less as well as my peers, but because I'd left India at age four, I couldn't read or write it. However, I would have been behind my classmates regardless, because the Indian elementary school system is far ahead of the American. Worst of all, I would have no summer break and I would be the new girl yet again.

Moving between India and the States brought changes that left me perpetually confused and feeling like an outsider. For one, I couldn't keep my spellings straight—in the U.S. I'd write "colour" and "flavour," and in India, "color" and "flavor." Then there were more embarrassing cultural mix-ups. In the U.S., wearing a tank top to deal with heat was perfectly normal, but the same outfit in India came off as wildly provocative, drawing snickers from my cousins and *tut-tuts* from my uncles. Deeper than that, I was always missing some important event of pop culture or rite of passage that my peers had experienced, because I was in the wrong country. I didn't wholly identify with the collective experiences of children in either place. I had one foot in each culture, but no firm footing in either of them.

At the time, the school consisted of just a few square rooms topped with thatched roofs, standing in a dusty courtyard surrounded by neem trees. It was in the Adyar neighborhood, near the Aavin Milk Bar, a major landmark in seventies Madras, where so many families took their kids for shakes or sticks of frozen milk. Located at the intersection of five roads, the Milk Bar was a round compound and was shaded by trees, providing lovers a safe place to furtively meet camouflaged by swarms of friends. It was also a place where young families could enjoy an inexpensive outing in the cool evening air. We always passed it on the way home from school and looked longingly at it like some sweet oasis.

Around 3:45 p.m. every weekday afternoon, the St. Michael's school bus spit me out, along with my cousin Rajni, below our little flat, always teeming with activity. In one room lived Rajni and her parents: my mother's younger brother Vichu and his wife, my aunt Bhanu. Once when I was three I tried to kill Rajni by stepping on her. Soon to arrive on the scene was her brother, Rohit, my main rival for my grandfather's affection. In the second bedroom were my two grandparents, me, and Neela, my mother's youngest sibling. As if that weren't enough, my cousin Aarti, my uncle Ravi's daughter, often came from Delhi to stay with us, too, as did Neela's cousin Vidya, the daughter of one of my grandmother's brothers. Add to that my grandfather's students, who, hoping to raise their exam scores, would loiter in the living room hall on Sundays. Needless to say, the time spent in my grandfather's flat stood in stark contrast to my life as a latch-key kid in the crowded metropolis of New York City.

Rajni and I arrived at a rare time of quiet in an otherwise bustling home. My grandparents were usually napping in their room. Once we washed our hands and feet and had a snack, we were encouraged to nap, too, at least until the sun sank and the temperature dipped. Whether we napped or not, we weren't allowed to go out in the sun until after 4:30 p.m. My grandmother thought we were already too dark from playing sports outside during school. You had only to read the matrimonial columns to see that light-skinned girls had it easier, even in a brown country like India. Indian culture was rife with color prejudice. Often the first word on the listing boasting of the eligible boy or girl for marriage would be "fair." "Wheatish" was used when they couldn't get away with saying "fair," and no one wanted to be called the euphemistic "dusky." Our time playing out-side during those summers was brief. We had only a couple of hours after 5:00 p.m. tiffin—the subcontinent's version of its colonizers' "tea," which brought *dosa* and *kachori* rather than cucumber sandwiches—to play fox hunt or a violent game of tag. Sometimes we'd build sand temples adorned with red and white hibiscus flowers, before darkness when the mosquitoes became too menacing.

The nights were so hot that most adults congregated on their veran-das, keeping an eye on us as we played. The sounds of our neighbors' lives blared through the neighborhood or colony almost as loudly as the TVs (which we ourselves only acquired in 1977). From our spots in the sand, we'd occasionally hear laughter or crying or the crack of an open hand connecting with soft flesh. Corporal punishment was the disciplinary tool of preference. I don't ever remember being grounded or having a privilege taken away. I had none to confiscate.

At times, we kids in the colony all seemed to function as a large, unofficial family. Often we would stop playing to find the closest door and bang on it, begging for water, until someone answered. With a sigh, some unlucky woman would bring out a pitcher and tumbler, which no doubt emptied out her small fridge's supply for the night, and watch as we all took greedy slugs. In a drought-ridden country like India, it was very bad form to refuse anyone water, and we children knew this. So those who lived on the ground floors of the apartment complexes often became de facto water coolers.

The close proximity in which people lived in India was in stark contrast to my independent existence in America. Here, everyone knew one another's business, and in general personal space and privacy were ephemeral. For naps, I always chose a spot on the cool green marble floor close to the side of the bed where my grandfather, or KCK as he was called, slept. It was that same spot my grandmother favored in rare moments of quiet. I watched his large, bearlike belly, barely covered by his undershirt, rise and fall. You could time a clock to the sound of his gentle snoring. I'd often wait for the sounds of his waking: the familiar clearing of his throat, a grumble, and a mumble. He'd open one eye, peer down at me, and whisper, so as not to rouse my grandmother, a notoriously light sleeper, still asleep beside him. "Psst, eh, Pads?" he'd say. "There's a two-rupee note in my bush shirt pocket hanging there. What say you go to All-In-One and grab a little something for you and me?"

The All-In-One was the first store to sprout up among the colony flats, the Indian version of the many bodegas and Korean delis that define daily life in New York. The All-In-One was the size of a small single-car garage. It sold shaving cream, laundry detergent, plastic wastepaper baskets and buckets for bathing, the disinfectant Dettol, bandages, medicines from Valium to aspirin to asthma inhalers, scissors, paper, pencils, copybooks, savory snacks, chocolates, and Rasna, a powdered drink mix similar to Tang—most of it kept under a glass counter or behind it in a glass cabinet. There were little jars of candies and biscuits and five-paise (about one-twentieth of a rupee) packs of Chiclets. There were two coolers, one for soft-drink bottles and the other, a metal icebox, for Popsicles and ice cream. In the back of the All-In-One, jute sacks of rice, sugar, lentils, coffee, and other raw goods lay heaped behind an iron scale. Two round iron plates hung from the ceiling by chains attached to a bar. The clanging sound the plates made as goods were measured and sold was ear-piercing in intensity. I made anywhere from three to eight trips a day to the All-In-One. I could be dispatched there for oil by my grandmother or for a notebook by Neela, or accompany my uncle Ravi when he was in town and went to buy cigarettes on the sly, bribing me with cold Indian sodas or Cadbury Dairy Milk chocolate bars.

My postnap trips to the store were always clandestine. After instructing me to fish out the rupee notes from his shirt pocket, my grandfather would put a finger to his lips. I knew I had to remove his shirt from the hook by the cupboard without jingling any change that may have been resting in its pockets. I had to take the amount he instructed and slip out of the room. Even if I'd succeeded in not waking my grandmother, I still had to elude inquiries from my busybody aunt Bhanu, who, if not napping in her own room with her daughter, Rajni, would be in the kitchen preparing for five o'clock tea and tiffin.

I never bothered to fish out my *chapals* (slippers) from the shoe closet by the front door, because the sliding wooden doors made too much noise.

And anyway, our whole street was sand. The rest of the neighborhood kids and I played barefoot. But the main road was tarred. At that time of day, with the sun high in the sky and my path baking under the Coromandel heat, walking briskly, let alone casually strolling, would mean second-degree burns. But if I ran as fast as I could, literally hotfooting it, I could just about endure until I reached the cool relief of the All-In-One's stone floor to complete my task. I was to buy two single-serving vanilla ice cream cups, one for me and one for KCK.

He loved those little cups, each with a wooden spoon taped to the bottom. I usually had enough change to buy myself a small packet of rose mints, Pez-shaped baby-pink candies with a mild but distinct flavor and light floral scent. On the way home I carried the two cups in one hand and the mints and change in the other. I tried to run even faster, because in addition to suffering the scalding tarred road and maintaining the secret of my mission, I had to contend with the melting ice cream. KCK and I ate the cups of ice cream quietly in the bedroom while my grandma slept, beaming at each other between bites, the lovely pain of cold in our mouths.

When I went out for my mission, I always left the front door slightly ajar, barely noticeable to the passing eye, so I could easily sneak back in. It almost always worked. Once, though, Aunt Bhanu caught me upon my return as the door squeaked open. "Eh?! What were you doing outside in the sun?" She seemed really mad, as if I'd stolen from her purse. Just then my grandfather cleared his throat loudly and called out for her to bring him tea.

"Pads just came in from somewhere, Tha-Tha!" she tattled. "She's left the door open and gone without telling anyone. Now she has something in her hands and all!"

"It's fine, Bhanu, I asked her to fetch me a stamp from All-In-One." Perhaps the *only* thing All-In-One did not sell was stamps. "I told her to get a little something for herself. Send her here, I'll deal with the child. And bring me my chai please, my throat is bothering."

Bhanu knew my grandfather was never short of stamps, given his weekly trips to the post office for his pension checks, but she also knew never to cross her father-in-law. I slid sheepishly past her and into the bedroom. The commotion of course had roused my grandmother, lying in the bed. As soon as we put wooden spoon to paper cup, she said, without moving or even opening her eyes, "Will you please stop putting that child up to no good!"

Rajima kept a low profile and rarely contradicted her husband outside of the bedroom. But in the privacy of that room, from our place on the floor, Neela and I heard her speak her mind. We learned who really held the seat of power in our family.

I wouldn't understand until years later why my errand caused such a row between two loving and mild-mannered people. KCK was diabetic. *Severely* so. And he was afflicted with a mighty sweet tooth. He'd need one to love the vast array of saccharine Indian sweets, which he did but which I decidedly do not. He adored *ladoos* and *jalebis* and *payasams* laced with cardamom and cashews in thick, sweet milk. *Payasams* I didn't mind, but only as an adult have I come to like *ladoos*, tiny balls of deep-fried chickpea-flour batter mixed with nuts and raisins and bound by syrup into large balls. I still feel sick after eating the traffic-cone-orange *jalebis*, sugary dough extruded into hot, saffron-spiked oil.

Fortunately for me, he didn't stop at these traditional confections. He also kept a sleeve of Marie biscuits hidden behind the volumes on his bookshelf. He'd snack on them, I'm sure, but he'd also dole them out as treats for us kids. Occasionally, when a burst of affection for us overtook him or when one of his students did well on a quiz, he'd produce a biscuit, as if out of nowhere, as a reward.

KCK taught me to make the first dessert I ever even considered replicating myself: a simple cold *payasam* of mashed bananas, milk, sugar, and cinnamon or cardamom. I have always preferred salty, tangy, crunchy things to sweets, especially the aggressively sugary Indian sweets, but for him I would have eaten all the *ladoos* and *jalebis* in Madras. My grandmother allowed me to make banana *payasam* for the *prasadam* that accompanied the religious ceremonies we marked at home.

The flavors I loved most were the tart, sour notes in things like green mango and tamarind. Before school, my new best friends—P., K., and C.—and I would sit under a tamarind tree on the campus of St. Michael's Academy. From its shade, we'd watch Mrs. Balagopal, my plump, smiling third-grade teacher, arrive on her scooter, her colorful, wildly printed sari fluttering behind her like a superhero's cape. I'd look for D., a boy who lived in my neighborhood. He was taller than the others and a great cricket player to boot.

Every so often, as a strong breeze shook the boughs of the tamarind trees, we'd hear a rustling and pods would tumble through the lacy leaves and fall to the ground. Sometimes they would hit us as they fell. When they're brown and ripe, the papery pods contain sweet, tangy flesh clinging to stone-like seeds, but as kids we'd also eat them when they were still green. My grandmother loved these young pods, still seedless, crisp and tart like green mango. "*Kanna,* there are some nice *imli* pods at your school," she'd remind me. "Knock a few down and bring them back in your school bag." If none fell on their own, I'd chuck stones at the tree.

The silky rustling of tamarind leaves always reminded me of the rustling of my grandmother's sari. Women in my family keep their bodies hidden, their breasts and bellies concealed even from their children and husbands. Only after my grandmother had cleaned up with Bhanu, turned off the lights, and put everyone to sleep would she dare creep through the bedroom, past me and Neela, to change her sari. I'd hear her unwrapping herself from six yards of fabric, the colorful silk and the folds of her body invisible in the darkness. I'd hear her searching her sari for the rupees that she kept tied in a small bundle of fabric at the end, a sort of makeshift pocket. Indian women hide many things in their saris: keys, extra safety pins, loose change, gemstones. In the seventies, some women, though certainly not Jima, even hid hashish to be smuggled through customs in a compartment sewn into the bottom hem. Sometimes as she undressed and shook out her sari a secret bundle would strike me or Neela, just like those falling tamarind pods. We would try to stifle our giggles. We knew that, even though we couldn't see it, she was exposed. At the time our only response to this advanced screening of womanhood was laughter.

In that room late at night, I'd also sometimes hear an urgent murmuring that I never quite understood to be what I know now it was: the quiet pleas of my grandfather, trying to get frisky in the dark. The forced proximity of our lives meant an intense physical closeness. When I was scared by a nightmare, I'd find my whimpering soothed by the arm of my grandfather reaching down to envelop me from his bed.

I was still a girl, unaware of the real meanings and intimacies of adulthood. Yet I did know where the answers to many of those mysteries were kept: inside the Godrej. Godrej was the brand of armoire we and nearly everyone else had, and just as the word "Kleenex" stands in for tissue, "Godrej" came to refer to the armoire itself. Technically, the house had four Godrejs. Yet only one mattered: the one in my grandparents' room. Narrow and made of heavy steel, it looked like a locker with two doors, one with a squeaky handle above a keyhole and the other with a long mirror. If we kids heard a jangling of keys or the creaking of a metal door, we'd all come running, hoping to get a glimpse inside. Occasionally I'd loiter near the Godrej, like a cat beneath the dinner table, waiting for my chance. From my sporadic peeks into its interior, I pieced together a map of its contents. I knew the shelves were lined with old newspaper. On those shelves were piles of my grandfather's bush shirts, buttoned-down, four-pocketed garments in plaid, simple prints, and polished cotton. He had about fifty and wore about three. His Rolleiflex camera was there, along with the black-and-white photos he took with it. The Godrej also contained my grandmother's wedding sari, an ornately brocaded blue-and-black Benares silk, heavy with gold-threaded embroidery at the hem. My favorite of all her saris was a florid Technicolor blue-and-purple double-shaded thick silk with gold embroidery threaded throughout the body as well as the border.

My grandfather kept the keys to the Godrej—a set of five, each with a different number written on its bow—in his breast pocket. When he napped in the afternoon, he'd slip the set under his pillow. Occasionally, I noticed my grandmother extract a set from under her sari. I was never sure whether there were two sets or one. When you asked one of them, the other one had the keys. Or they weren't sure where they were. This might have been deliberate, a sleight of hand.

I did know that there was one key that only my grandmother possessed. Because within this chamber of secrets was another, a drawer to which my grandmother alone had access. This key hung on her *thali,* a sort of necklace that Hindu husbands tie around the necks of their wives to mark the marriage. They can be elaborate and bejeweled or as simple as a cord or string with an ornament attached. I admired my grandmother's, a braided gold rope, as thick as a haricot vert, with gold beads and two flat, square charms with forked bottoms and an insignia welded into the center of each. Yet part of me can't help but see the *thali* as a way to claim property, a beautiful dog collar. You almost expect that if you were to look closely, you'd find in small print, "If found, please return to . . ." I suppose you could say the same of a wedding ring, though both spouses wear those.

As they did with many aspects of the female South Indian uniform, women found ways to employ the *thali* for quotidian convenience. Some kept safety pins on their *thalis,* in case someone lost a button or a young girl needed help fastening her sari. Like the contents of the Godrej, the keys and the ornaments of the *thali* were often invisible to me, hidden as they were in my grandmother's cavernous cleavage or tucked between her sari and blouse.

I'm not sure even my grandfather knew what was in that drawer. And I'm not sure he cared. But I did. From my prowling, I knew that it contained her good jewelry, my grandfather's watches, his beloved tortoiseshell fountain pen, and our passports, along with other important documents. There were letters, too, from dead relatives, or aerogrammes from my mother in America, detailing her life and other things she observed in her new culture that I had yet to face. I was not allowed to read them, but my mom's letters were read to me often. The drawer also contained all the beauty-related goodies, from powder puffs to perfume, that I'd ferried from the U.S. in my suitcase. These had to be kept from me and Neela, otherwise we'd burn through them during our Kabuki-appropriate grooming sessions. My grandmother wore very little makeup. Most days, she swiped the rim of each eye with a paste of homemade black kohl, rubbing any excess into her hair. If I was lucky enough to be nearby when she opened the drawer on the day of an occasion worthy of a little more primping, I might get more than a peek. She'd sometimes call me over as she applied her powder, and I'd stand at her knees while the powder fell around me like snow.

The birth of my cousin Rohit, Rajni's brother and the spawn of Aunt Bhanu and Uncle Vichu, did little to weaken the female stranglehold on our home. We vastly outnumbered the men. The main activity of the women in my household was cooking or preparing to cook. We'd all gather on the floor of the dining room or kitchen while the men sat reading the paper on the veranda at the end of the day. My grandmother sat hunched over an old wood coconut grater, an *aruvamanai,* steadying the wooden block with her knee as she scraped the fruit against its perpendicular blade and white shavings fell onto a plate underneath. My aunts trimmed, peeled, and sliced potatoes—always in their palms, not on a cutting board. I sat transfixed, more so by the display than the food. While these quietly focused women bent over to do their work, the ends, or *pallus*, of their saris dipped down and the world was revealed to me. Indian women were extremely demure and rarely showed any skin. To get a glimpse of their mysterious cleavage was very unusual. It meant they had their guard down, or that they had accepted you into their female coven. One day, I watched the same ritual of cutting vegetables before the cooking started at my great-aunt Chinnu's house. Her housekeeper, Kalyani, was a dark-skinned, thickly built woman (today she'd be considered a brick house), and that day as she chopped, I caught a glimpse of her breasts jiggling as the sharp smell of green chilies tickled my nose. I remember feeling a quiver in my stomach, an almost sexual thrill. Later, when Kalyani had her first child, she would let me watch as she breast-fed in the storeroom.

In the kitchen, my grandmother wielded a large iron ladle, blackened over time and permanently greasy at the base of its long handle, which she used for frying (for some reason called "tempering" in Indian recipes) black mustard seeds and other spices. First, she poured oil into the ladle, then held it over the stovetop flame. When the oil was good and hot, she added mustard seeds, dried red chilies, then curry leaves and a pounded, powdered resin called asafoetida. The distinct smell of mustard seeds and asafoetida frying, along with that of curry leaves, is what distinguishes southern from northern Indian food to me. The popping seeds also act as a sort of low-tech timer to tell you when the spices are sufficiently roasted. At the first crackle and pop, my grandmother would whisk the ladle away and add the oil mixture to whatever dish she was making. We all knew to stay clear of that scalding-hot ladle, with its contents smoking. If we were particularly hungry and stalking her like vultures, we'd cut a wide path around her until she delivered those spices to a pot of food. The familiar hushed sizzle, like the sound of a hot pan placed in a sink full of water, meant it was about time to eat.

This ritual would immediately precede the serving of many dishes, such as *rasam*, a thin soup made with tamarind; *sambar*, a soupy lentil stew; or, my favorite, *thayir sadam*, a cool, savory porridge of salted yogurt and rice. *Thayir sadam* is the ultimate South Indian comfort food. The anytime treat costs pennies to make and fills you up, thanks to a healthy combo of protein and carbs. It would be ladled into our lunch boxes during the winter months. In the hot season, it would be dinner, eaten after we returned home, sweaty from playing down the lane.

Every housewife had her own special concoction that she mixed into yogurt rice. My mom fried freshly minced ginger and green chilies; my aunt added fresh pomegranate seeds and chopped cilantro; and others served it plain with just a spoonful of fiery Indian pickles made from green mango, sorrel, or lime. Few versions were anything but comforting and delightful, though my grandmother had the magic touch. With the contents of her iron ladle—mustard seeds and the like, plus perhaps crunchy fried lentils or even pieces of lotus root cured with spices, dried in the sun, and brought over from my grandfather's village, Palghat, in Kerala—she would turn rice and yogurt into a meal that half a dozen kids would greedily lick from their cupped fingers. You'd smell the spices frying or hear the mustard seeds popping and know: T-minus a few minutes to *thayir sadam*. When there was plenty of yogurt, the dish was creamy and thick. When there wasn't and she stretched the yogurt with milk and water, it was liquid and thin.

In India, yogurt is almost always homemade. It's easy, really. My aunts would boil milk (raw and unhomogenized), let it cool to room temperature, and add a bit of yesterday's yogurt, the starter reserved for this purpose. They'd cover the mixture and let it sit overnight, until the cultures did their work and the milk soured and thickened. Because each batch of new yogurt contains some of yesterday's yogurt, and because this process happens daily for many years, "yesterday" is sort of a misnomer. The yogurt used to start each new batch is, in essence, many years old itself and becomes a kind of family property. Young brides, for instance, will take a spoonful of their mother's yogurt to their marital home.

My grandmother would set her yogurt in a "quiet" part of the kitchen. As my culinary universe expanded, I assumed that this "quiet" suggested some delicate process at work, one similar to the rising of a soufflé, which French chefs semi-jokingly request that you not disturb by talking while it is in the oven. Yet now I'm sure she meant "quiet," as in a place where none of us kids would disturb it with our jostling and shoving. I was the worst, she tells me. I would routinely knock over the yogurt as I climbed up to reach for the pickle jars above the counter. To keep it safe, she moved it farther back, into the darker part of the kitchen counter. I assumed that the darkness also somehow assisted in the yogurt-making process. But it was really just about keeping the yogurt safe. You see, there were lizards lurking in the dark and I was scared of them. Or, as my grandmother says, "The lizards were quietly guarding the curds for me."

Her strategy might have kept me away from the yogurt, but I still spent plenty of time in the kitchen and the attached storeroom where larger amounts of surplus pickles were kept. On the top pantry shelf, above the jute sacks of rice and lentils and drums of sliced dried lotus root, was a row of glass jars containing a deliriously tempting array of pickles. In the kitchen, there were just a few varieties, but here they taunted me with their number. There were green-mango pickles, lime pickles, and ginger pickles. There were pickles made from young jackfruit, sorrel, tamarind, gooseberry, and red chilies stuffed with cumin and fennel seeds. These Indian pickles were much more complex than the vinegary pickled vegetables in the West. They were pickled in mustard oil or sesame oil, with

yogurt rice

Serves 8 to 10

5 cups cooked white Basmati rice
4 cups plain whole-milk yogurt
1½ teaspoons salt
2 cups peeled and diced English cucumbers or 2 cups fresh pomegranate
    seeds
¼ cup canola oil
2 tablespoons white gram lentils (urad dal, found at Indian grocery stores)
2 teaspoons black mustard seeds
½ teaspoon asafoetida powder (found at Indian grocery stores)
1 to 2 medium serrano chilies with seeds, diced, or more to taste
1 dozen fresh medium curry leaves, torn into small pieces

In a large bowl, combine the rice, yogurt, and salt, kneading them together
with your hands. Then stir in the cucumber (in spring and summer) or the
pomegranate seeds (in fall and winter). Set aside.

In a small sauté pan, heat the canola oil over medium heat. After a few
minutes, when the oil is hot and shimmering, add in the lentils. When they're
just beginning to turn golden (after about 3 minutes), add in the mustard seeds
and asafoetida powder. Stir briefly. You will hear a popping sound when the
mustard seeds begin to cook.

After just a minute, when the popping becomes more frequent, add in the
chilies and curry leaves. Stir for 1 to 2 minutes, then remove the pan from heat.

Pour the lentil-mustard oil over the rice mixture and stir well with a spoon.

This dish should be served at room temperature or cold, and it's great
for a summer lunch or dinner. If you're making it ahead, just stir in a bit of
water to loosen it up before serving; it should have a porridge- or oatmeal-like
consistency.

fenugreek and all sorts of spices mixed in a certain order in a certain proportion that changed with the whim and preference of my grandmother. When relatives came from Kerala or Tanjore or my uncle Ravi visited from Delhi, we were brought pickles from other regions my grandparents maintained a hankering for.

I couldn't resist their siren song and once, in the quiet of the afternoon, I set out to make them mine with disastrous results. I was a good climber, still too small to be burdened by my weight, so up I went, from shelf to shelf like a temple monkey. When I was close enough, I stretched to grab a jar and, slick with oil, it slipped from my grasp and shattered. Glass and turmeric-yellow oil were everywhere. Too afraid to call out and summon my angry aunt Bhanu, too afraid of the broken glass to descend, I froze there, hanging on to the ledge for what seemed like ten minutes before Neela opened the door and rescued me.

In the summer, as long as the yogurt survived our rambunctiousness, we would often gather around Rajima on the cool green marble floor in a semicircle and she'd place in front of each of us a little steel bowl called a *katori*. She presided over a larger steel bowl filled with leftover rice from the big brass pot that was always on the stove. She would mix cool yogurt into the rice with her right hand while turning the bowl with her left. I can still hear its tinny scrape against the marble floor. Bhanu would bring the iron ladle, bend down, and pour in the oil mixture as Rajima continued to mix. She would then take turns dropping wet dollops of rice into our upturned and outstretched hands. If you hadn't eaten your portion by the time she came around to you again, she'd place the next dollop in your bowl. If you let these pile up, the older kids like Neela or Vidya would snatch your bowl and empty it into their mouths right under your nose.

As we ate, she told us stories and fables: the story of the sparrow and the king; tales of mischievous Lord Krishna, who, as a child, stole butter, pulled girls' plaits, and bit every apple on a tree only once, wasting the fruit for everyone else; and, my favorite, the fable of the cunning myna bird, who laid its eggs in a crow's nest while the crow was away hunting. Because myna eggs and crow eggs looked the same, the crow would be none the wiser. And while the poor crow sat dutifully on the eggs until they hatched, and then cared for the chicks, the myna enjoyed itself, flying in the moonlight and singing in the trees. Once the myna chicks were old enough to fly and be recognized as imposters, they'd leave and join their parents for a carefree life.

In the courtyard of our complex, there was a big flat-leafed tree with white trumpet flowers that shaded all the flats. From our veranda, Neela and Rajni and Rohit and I would gaze at the crows' nests in the tree. Over the years, we watched many generations of crows hatch and grow. We watched many myna birds perch and sing. I'd often stake out one of the nests, waiting to catch a sneaky myna laying her eggs. Every summer when I returned from high school in the States, an amateur photography buff, I trained my telephoto lens on those little hungry open mouths, trying to identify the Trojan chicks. I wondered then if my grandmother had invented the story as a metaphor. Perhaps she, too, wished she could fly away, just for a while, to escape the relentless duties of family. Instead she was stuck nesting on the marble floor in front of her bowl, surrounded by so many little brown hands outstretched.

Of the two of my aunts who lived in the house in Madras's Besant Nagar neighborhood, my aunt Bhanu was older than Neela by several years, so she took on the maternal role of enforcer and delouser. It was Bhanu who enrolled me in St. Michael's and poor Bhanu who was called into the head office to meet with Brother, the scowling headmaster who kept admonishing her to rein in her low-performing American niece.

It was Bhanu who locked us together in her room until I mastered my lessons. It was Bhanu who treated us with the Indian equivalent of RID whenever we kids came back from school scratching our heads like mangy dogs. Once, I had both exams *and* lice. Again, Bhanu locked me away. Just beyond her door, I could hear the others laughing and Doordarshan blaring on our TV. The state-run network that was our only channel played clips of songs from Bollywood movies like music videos, all in a row. It was the equivalent of American kids gathering in front of the TV to watch *American Bandstand* or *Soul Train* on the weekends. Meanwhile I was trapped in Bhanu's room, my head stinging and stinking as she meticulously scraped my scalp to raw dermis with a double-sided fine-tooth comb, while simultaneously drilling me on my multiplication tables.

Without Bhanu, I would never have learned the Secret of the Nines (9, 18, 27, 36, 45 . . . the digits always add up to nine) or be able to balance my checkbook. As a kid, I thought I hated Bhanu. Now, I can only hope that I'm able to tame and care for my daughter the way Bhanu did me. More concerned with results than our affection, she was totally fine with her status as least favorite aunt. Today I am immensely grateful for what was clearly great love, but back then I resented her for what I saw as unnecessary punishment and arbitrary cruelty, and, even worse, for birthing Rajni, the only threat to my supreme reign as house cutie.

While Aunt Bhanu played the role of stern authority figure, Neela—technically my aunt but only seven years my senior—played my sisterly conspirator. Neela and I were thick as thieves then. And after all these years, in health and sickness, through kids and divorce, we still are. Rather than medicating my scalp, like Bhanu, Neela braided my hair. Instead of wrestling me into uniforms, she dressed me in her colorful hand-me-downs. Neela and I acquired a nickname. Older relatives would often call both of us *alangari,* which in Tamil means one who likes to dress up or beautify herself. It was their way of chiding us for not paying the same close attention to our studies as we did to our appearance. We didn't care. When I was really young, around three, Neela and her cousin Vidya used to dress me as a boy. They even drew a mustache on me with eyebrow pencil. From an early age, I got good at doing makeup. Neela was my first client. A few years later, I started plucking my mother's eyebrows for allowance money. Even today my mother demands my services whenever I see her. She still offers my usual five-dollar fee.

The only thing Neela and I loved more than making each other up was snacking. Near St. Michael's was a stand that sold softball-sized potato-filled samosas, expertly fried and spiced. The samosa, of course, is India's answer to the empanada or, as the former Lower East Sider in me must add, the knish. The outside of the samosa, however, is even flakier than those others, made as it is with plenty of ghee, or clarified butter. This makes the samosa even worse for you than its doughy Western counterparts and also even more delicious. Then there were *kachori*, another member of the stuffed-and-fried family. At home, we were more likely to eat *aloo tikkis*, which are sort of like samosas without the flaky jacket. Aunt Bhanu was the *tikki* master of Madras. For my eighth birthday, she deftly formed what seemed like hundreds of potato patties before breading and frying them in a shallow pool of oil. When I had my first McDonald's hash brown, I thought to myself, *This is a very poor* aloo tikki.

Only on special occasions did my family make these types of treats at home, because the process made the entire house smell like frying oil and because they took a houseful of laborers to make. For instance, when we made the crunchy snacks called *murukku*, the women of my family would gather at Chinnu's house and converge on an old bedsheet in the hall. With oil on our hands, we'd handle the rice and lentil flour dough, simultaneously twisting the dough with our fingers as we formed spirals on the sheet. (For both the helix created by the twisting and the resulting shape, we called this all-day operation "spinning *murukku*.") Then we laid each spiral on the sheet to dry before Bhanu fried them all. Before we started the spinning, of course, we always molded a knob of dough into a rudimentary figure, dabbed near the head with red vermillion powder, meant to represent Lord Ganesh, the gluttonous god who adored snacking. I'm no expert on the standards and practices of Hinduism, but my guess is that this figure served as a talisman, ensuring that the *murukku* would turn out well.

At home, Neela and I conducted many experiments to clone the pleasure of *ampapads*—a sort of fruit leather made from mango that can only be found in the north. Though *ampapads* can be sour (*khatta*) or sweet (*meeta*), both Neela and I liked the sour ones most. Whenever my beloved uncle Ravi visited from New Delhi, he'd bring what seemed like suitcases full of *ampapads*. We'd suck wads of the stuff all day, like ballplayers with chew, at least until my grandmother or Aunt Bhanu caught us and insisted we stop lest we get stomachaches. Our attempts at producing homemade *ampapads* were destined to fail, of course, because making *ampapads* at home would be like replicating Fruit Roll-Ups in your kitchen without a dehydrator. Still, we'd smash and press and finally, tired of wasting good fruit, give up, instead simply dousing the fruit with salt, chili powder, and lime juice. Often we'd bring bowls of our concoctions to eat on the veranda, our bare legs splayed on the marble, cold from the shade of the big tree.

We also loved *churan*, intensely flavored powders or tiny balls, especially *jeera goli* (spheres made from ingredients like black salt and cumin) and our favorite, *anar dana* (made from dried pomegranate seeds and spices). There were many kinds of *churan*, which are mostly used to settle the stomach after a heavy meal. They are bracingly sour and salty with a touch of sweetness, and so intense they make the sides of your mouth twinge with expectation at first sight, let alone first bite. They are meant to be eaten in small doses, but Neela and I often made whole meals of *churan*, popping *golis* into our mouths like Raisinets.

Once in a while we burned a wok trying to make our *churan*, and Jima, Bhanu, or another matriarch would banish us from the kitchen.

"You should've told us," they'd say. "We would've helped you." *You're not getting it,* Neela and I thought. *This is our party and you're not invited.* To this day, the elder women of my household in Chennai still regard Neela or me with suspicion whenever we enter the kitchen to make anything other than tea. No matter that I host a cooking show or that Neela has raised two healthy daughters who clearly haven't starved or been disfigured by a kitchen accident.

Of course, we never went long after a reprimand before returning to the kitchen, especially in the quiet of midafternoon, when the napping gatekeepers left it unguarded. Like janitors in a lab, we waited out the scientists until we were alone with the chemicals and could tinker. We made many versions of chili cheese toast, a classic Indian snack that today is on every hotel menu in India. The formula for this subcontinental club sandwich is bread, butter, cheese, and minced green chilies. At the time, we used Britannia brand bread, a knockoff Wonder Bread (the packaging even sported colorful squares instead of circles), which was like a scratchy motel pillow compared with the soft, fluffy down of the real thing. We used Amul brand "cheese"—or, more accurately, processed cheese-like product, because it had all the quality of Laughing Cow wedges left out too long without the wrapper. But no matter. Decked out with minced chilies or Maggi brand Hot & Sweet—essentially ketchup and Tabasco swirled into one—the sandwich never disappointed. We cooked it with a sort of pie iron, a contraption with two long wood-covered handles, like those of scissors, which opened and closed the metal encasement. We'd hold a stick of butter like a marker and scribble the fat on the inside of the metal, then close it around the sandwich and hold it over the stovetop flame, turning it until the bread was a crunchy shell for the molten, processed goodness inside.

On the side, we ate cucumber slices topped with a tart spice mixture called *chaat masala.* We ate the cucumbers with toothpicks—we thought the toothpicks made us very sophisticated. We also made chocolate milk-shakes to go with the sandwiches, which were basically Cadbury Drinking Chocolate powder swirled into milk. We would hide our small tumblers behind all the food in the fridge so no one would even know they were there, until everyone went to sleep at night, and then we would have our midnight feast. It was hard to get any private time in that house without several generations watching your every move. So our little midnight parties were just for us older kids, no adults, no Rajni or Rohit.

Most of all, Neela and I loved the category of snacks called *chaat*. *Chaat* comes in such vast variety that only the few qualities every example shares—namely, a thrilling mixture of temperatures, textures (crunchy, crispy, and soft in all of their own myriad degrees), and flavors (hot, sweet, tart, and tangy)—can provide a meaningful definition. *Chaat*, to me, succeeds via culinary chemical principle: the combustion generated by opposites brought together in a bowl. Though things have changed, when I was a kid, no restaurant with four walls and self-respect would sell *chaat*. The pleasures and thrills offered by *chaat* were the domain of street vendors, operating out of stalls or pushcarts. The best were composed in front of you, in Delhi. Our beloved *chaatwallah*, near India Gate, made an exceptional version of my favorite, *papri chaat*: crunchy fried semolina discs dressed with warm chickpeas and potatoes, spice powders like red chili and black cumin, and the holy trinity of *chaat* sauces—tart, cooling yogurt; bright cilantro-and-mint green chili chutney; and tangy tamarind-date chutney. Those three sauces could create *chaat* from little else—potato, crunchy chickpea-flour noodles, an exploded samosa—resulting in an elegant hodgepodge, an incredibly complex-tasting dish.

Whenever I visited Delhi to see my uncle Ravi, I made him stop for *chaat* on the way home from the airport, perhaps for *pani puri* (or *golgappa*, as it's also called). This meant watching the *chaatwallah* pull a miniature sphere of *puri* (bread that's fried so it puffs and becomes crunchy) from a pile, poke a hole in its top with his finger, and add a dollop of potatoes, black chickpeas, and tamarind-date chutney inside. Then he'd dunk the whole thing in *pani,* which looks like swamp water but is actually a strange and beguiling mix of pureed mint, chili, tamarind, spices, and water. You'd knock it back in one exhilarating bite. Nowadays, you're often presented with the components and required to assemble each bite yourself, which is a bit like your favorite chef presenting you with his *mise en place* of prepped ingredients. *Pani puri* is never as good as when a master makes it.

What Neela and I craved in particular about *chaat* was the unique flavor that defined and united the array of snacks. We knew this as *chaatpati.* Think of it as the Indian umami. When a snack combined saltiness, tartness, sweetness, and spiciness in that magical, mouth-smacking proportion, then that snack had *chaatpati.* At the time, we had no words to describe that sought-after sensation, so when asked to explain, we'd say, "You know, *tlck tlck,*" as we clicked our tongues against the roofs of our mouths, the sound of satisfaction. For us, *chaatpati* was the condition to which all food should aspire. For me, that has pretty much remained the case for my whole life. As a high school student and lapsed vegetarian, I became enamored of the Double Bacon Western Cheeseburger at Carl's Jr., because the combination of salty bacon, creamy melted cheese, and sweet, piquant barbecue sauce amounted to *chaatpati.* Given the crunchy onion ring that topped the patty, I was basically eating a *chaat* burger. When I'd eat my beloved nachos from Green Burrito, I was drawn to the *chaat*-like qualities—there were chips (some crunchy, some soggy) as well as tart, spicy salsas and cooling dollops of sour cream. Had there been a sweet component, the nachos might have officially reached *chaatpati* status.

Even as a young girl I could tell that the South Indian chutneys we ate on the streets of Chennai were more balanced and round than the jagged-edged northern ones we had eaten in Delhi. We missed their sharpness, and often when we were hungry or bored, we set out to re-create it. Our best sauce to come of all those years of trial and error was our *chaatpati* tamarind-date chutney. This dark and gooey sludge became my first mother sauce of sorts, because it instantly woke up any bland or boring ingredient and made it finger-sucking good.

When Neela and I cooked, we were as obsessed with reproducing that tang and tingle as we were with replicating Sharmila Tagore's eyeliner in

chaatpati chutney

Makes 1½ cups

¼ cup natural tamarind concentrate (I prefer bottled Laxmi brand)
2 teaspoons ground cumin
2 teaspoons ground coriander
1 to 2 teaspoons cayenne powder, to taste
20 dates (about 4½ ounces), pitted and finely chopped
2 teaspoons kosher salt

In a 2-quart saucepan, bring 4 cups water to a boil. Add the tamarind concentrate, cumin, coriander, cayenne, dates, and salt and gently boil over medium heat for 25 to 30 minutes, stirring constantly with a wooden spoon and mashing the dates to create a pulpy mixture. The finished chutney should look like a very loose jam or thick barbeque sauce.

the old Hindi movies we studied. Tagore was a great beauty. A Bengali actress who shot to prominence in art-house Satyajit Ray films, she then crossed over successfully into Bollywood and became a major leading-lady bombshell. In our favorite movie, *Amar Prem*, she plays a courtesan (which we did not even grasp the meaning of), and her appearance is slightly vulgar, with gaudy jewels, garish saris, and dime-sized *bindis*. This was our ideal. We admired this look the way my daughter lights up at the sight of any article of clothing in Katy Perry pink. Food and fashion were our twin passions, bound together in our feminine, Indian identities, even when we were young girls. Back then, eating was also a means of beautification, since the more *aloo tikki* and *murukku* you consumed, the more likely you'd reach a voluptuousness akin to an American size ten or twelve, required for looking good in a sari.

Indeed, food and femininity were intertwined for me from very early on. Cooking was the domain not of girls, but of women. You weren't actually allowed to cook until you mastered the basics of preparing the vegetables and dry-roasting and grinding the spices. You only assisted by preparing these *mise en places* for the older women until you graduated and were finally allowed to stand at the stove for more than boiling tea. Just as the French kitchens had their hierarchy of *sous-chefs* and *commis,* my grandmother's kitchen also had its own codes. The secrets of the kitchen were revealed to you in stages, on a need-to-know basis, just like the secrets of womanhood. You started wearing bras; you started handling the pressure cooker for lentils. You went from wearing skirts and half saris to wearing full saris, and at about the same time you got to make the rice-batter crepes called *dosas* for everyone's tiffin. You did not get told the secret ratio of spices for the house-made *sambar* curry powder until you came of marriageable age. And to truly have a womanly figure, you had to eat, to be voluptuously full of food.

This, of course, was in stark contrast to what was considered womanly or desirable in the West, especially when I started modeling. To look good in Western clothes you had to be extremely thin. Prior to this, I never thought about my weight except to think it wasn't ever enough. Then, with modeling, I started depending on my looks to feed myself (though my profession didn't allow me to actually eat very much). When I started hosting food shows, my career went from fashion to food, from not eating to really eating *a lot,* to put it mildly. Only this time the opposing demands of having to eat all this food and still look good by Western standards of beauty were off the charts. This tug-of-war was something I would struggle with for most of a decade.

chapter 5

Through the smoke and mirrors of television, my job looks like it's full of glamour and excitement. You'd be forgiven for thinking that all I do is show up in my designer dress, have a meal and a chat, and head home. And it's true, filming the show can be a thrill. *Top Chef* is a little like live sports—anything can happen. Plus there are knives and fire. But TV filming is comically slow. Lulls outnumber activity ten to one.

The long days of shooting—some end at midnight, some go even longer—are mostly downtime. But not good downtime. Strange downtime. Most of it is spent off the set in my dressing room, a small space overtaken by wardrobe racks. I have a single task during this time: not to mess up my hair, makeup, and clothes. I can't undo all of my glam squad's hard work just because I want to lie down. Or have a snack. Or, God forbid, blow my nose. At all times, I have about four people scrutinizing my every move. In that way, it's a little like spending time with my family.

Practically every movement I make requires a conversation. "She wants to sit down, should she keep the dress on?" Michelle, my makeup artist, might say. "It has a zip," says Albert, my stylist. "She should take it off." They talk about me like I'm not there, like two parents discussing their kid. My comfy jeans are not typically an option. Albert and Michelle won't allow it. The seams supposedly mark my legs. If Michelle had her way, rollers wouldn't leave my hair until a minute before I'm due on my mark. If Albert had his, I'd never sit down and, even better, would always wear my bathrobe, lest a wrinkle tarnish my dress.

Sometimes, all I want to do is shut my eyes, but a producer will come around to record lines that might need to be spliced into the show later. I'll get word that I'm finally due back on the set, so the producers will send a guy to mic me. But even once we do hustle to the set, we end up hanging around for a while. That's the way it goes during shooting: hurry up and wait. And often, during that waiting, I eat.

I eat at Judges' Table, even though we *never* eat at Judges' Table on the show. Not the contestants' food, mind you. Over the years, I have had many snacks on the set that are not competition food. In the old days it started with some innocent sliced apples with peanut butter; then in New Orleans, our returning judge Emeril Lagasse turned me on to a Thai take-out that brought noodles in coconut milk to the set. And even before that, I taught my on-set assistant (and *Top Chef*'s unsung hero), Jason, how to make an open-faced version of my childhood classic, the chili cheese toast. This started several years back, long before the hipster restaurant trend to put almost anything on a toasted slice of bread and charge upward of $12 for it. Back when I was growing up, chili cheese toast was a down-homey snack we made for teatime or when feeling peckish.

When you're tired and hungry, you just want something as decadent and rich as what the chefs give you, but without all the fancy stuff. You want something comforting. During shooting, my stomach seems to expand and expect to be fed copious amounts of food even when it doesn't need it.

The glacial pace of TV is to blame. On a Quickfire day, I try to eat a

chili cheese toast

Serves 1

2 to 3 serrano or other hot green chilies, minced
A squirt of fresh lemon juice
Salt to taste
Butter, softened
1 slice sourdough bread
1 slice Muenster or Monterey Jack cheese

Mix the chilies, lemon juice, and salt with a mortar and pestle, mashing together to create a relish.

Generously butter one side of the bread. Spread a heaping teaspoon of the chili relish on the other side of the slice. Top it with the cheese.

Toast the bread butter side down in a covered pan over medium heat. Cook for 2 to 3 minutes, then uncover and cook 1 minute more.

Remove the toast from the pan. Slice diagonally and garnish each triangle with a dollop of relish.

---

healthy breakfast, but after hair, makeup, and wardrobe, after getting to the set and going over the script, after the inevitable delays, six hours have passed and I'm ravenous. So when the contestants' food shows up, most of it made in true restaurant style, with more butter than a kilo of croissants, I eat more than I know I should. I probably eat every two hours when I'm on the set. Tom will sometimes ask, sipping a gin and tonic, "How can you possibly be hungry?" I tell him I can eat as much as he can drink.

I typically go for snacks that won't risk ruining my dress or makeup—you're welcome, Albert and Michelle. Some of the snacks are strange, creations inspired by whatever I spot in the fridge. Some of them become regulars in my rotation, like my latest pet concoction: cottage cheese doused in Cholula Hot Sauce. Sometimes I'll dunk chips or celery in it, like a dietetic version of ranch dip. I'm always trying to re-create some vaguely healthy version of junk food. You've got to have junk food. You've got to feel satisfied while still somehow keeping your waistline in check. This is the constant struggle that pervades my life. How do I look good and still be good at my job? How do I experience enough food so I know what I'm talking about on TV in the midst of these culinary heavyweights, and still look good while talking about it?

The men on the show have it easy, in part because men on TV have uniforms: There's the jacket, in black, blue, or gray. There's the shirt, the pants. I can never tell whether Tom is gaining or losing weight beneath his boxy suits. He always looks the same. Tom also has the benefit of being Tom, a decorated veteran of the restaurant kitchen. Like so many chefs, he is practiced at the taste-of-this, taste-of-that eating regimen. I'm the one who has to look like a glorified weathergirl, with formfitting dresses and all, which, don't get me wrong, I love—at least until I don't.

Unlike the other judges, who aren't there for the beginning two acts of the show, I have to gorge during the appetizer portion of the *Top Chef*–episode meal: the Quickfire. We're not a live show, but we sometimes function as one. We can't reshoot and reshoot; juicy rib eye steaks turn into cold meat and congealing fat. So the reality of the Quickfire is virtually identical to the way it appears on TV. Contestants are given a challenge on the spot—make an amuse-bouche using only products found in a vending machine; reinvent the po' boy sandwich—and forced to execute a dish without forethought or *mise en place.* The chefs must act on a combination of culinary instinct and creative impulse. Adrenaline shakes awake their true selves, and the food they produce reveals who they really are as cooks. I always come hungry. They deserve the full audience of my appetite. I stand with the episode's special guest, typically an established and celebrated chef, in front of a contestant and her dish, we eat, then we walk out of the frame. The cameras do a two-step around us and we walk back into frame in front of another contestant. The process is rapid fire: *Bite, bite, bite,* pause, adopt inscrutable facial expression, spew a vague comment that gives nothing away, and repeat. After a while my stomach begins to feel like a restaurant Dumpster. It was this kind of experience that made me devise a drink I call Cranberry Drano. I came up with it to help cleanse my digestive pipes after all the gluttonous eating on the show. During production I am likely to consume three full glasses of this potion a day, scrunching up my face the

cranberry drano

Serves 1

½ cup organic unsweetened 100% cranberry juice
1 tablespoon clear fiber powder
1 packet Emergen-C, or other vitamin C powder
1 cup still-hot green tea brewed with 1 teaspoon honey
4 to 5 ice cubes

Vigorously mix the cranberry juice, fiber powder, Emergen-C, and green tea in a tall tumbler. Add ice cubes. Drink immediately.

whole time, due to its less-than-pleasurable taste. (In spite of the taste, it gets me through to the other side of filming.)

During the Chicago season, the immoderation started with the very first Quickfire. The guest judge was Rocco DiSpirito. And this being Chicago, the contestants, all sixteen of them, were tasked with making deep-dish pizzas that showed off their culinary personalities. In other words, the already brawny deep-dishes were decked out with prosciutto and lamb sausage and duck, with oozy Taleggio and cream-filled burrata. In the interest of fairness, Rocco and I had to sample each one straight from the oven, then again later to see how it held up to delivery. Do the math: thirty-two tastes, several bites in each. And you can't take a small bite of deep-dish pizza—you cut off a bite with short length and width, but the height is fixed at, well, deep. I was in physical pain, devastated by my fullness.

By the filming of the second episode of the Chicago season, Darshan, my wardrobe diva at the time, noticed that my dress was tight. By the time the Chicago season wrapped, I had gained seventeen pounds. I felt horrible that I couldn't manage my job *and* my appearance. My divorce had just become final; I was living in hotels and had little control over what I ate even when I wasn't filming. That July, when I first moved into the Surrey, I had had the opposite problem. People wondered if I was possibly anorexic, because I couldn't eat from depression and was so thin. Mere months later, in November, after my divorce became final and I had filmed another season of *Top Chef,* I ballooned up two dress sizes. Every woman has a record of her body—a closet full of jeans and bras of various sizes, albums full of photographs revealing periods of weight gain and loss. I've also come to realize that as a fortysomething woman on TV, I'm a rapidly depreciating asset, like a car just driven off the lot. Then there's the added indignity of seeing my flaws dissected, zoomed in on, and gleefully mocked.

I've come to accept my weight gain as part of my *Top Chef* pact with the devil. But early on, I was in denial. To make sure we came in under budget, I used to suggest that we borrow clothes from designers. This is a common strategy for models and actresses, which gives onlookers the impression that they have bottomless closets. My stylist had to break it to me: to fit into clothes available for borrowing, I had to be a sample size—in other words, waiflike. I wasn't. By now, everyone on the set is used to my fluctuations. My beauty crew always finds a way to patch me up. From the start, Darshan would gather dresses in several sizes. She knew I'd jump up two or three sizes during filming. That, along with the magic of the camera—careful angling and long shots—helps hide the inevitable stomach paunch and back-of-the-arm pudge that always appear a few weeks in.

When I wasn't filming, I could control my weight fairly well through good eating habits and exercise, thanks to both a forgiving metabolism and a flexible schedule. What I could never control, however, was my skin. I hated the fact that my dark skin marked and mottled easily—from my mosquito bite–scarred legs, to the two pale circles on my left arm from the olden days of inoculations in India, to the scar on my right arm. I didn't love that my coloring set off the stretch marks behind my knees, which appeared during a teenage growth spurt, or those on my backside acquired from my many weight fluctuations. Various cuts and burns from cooking still remained, too, faded but nonetheless a reminder of every time I made some mistake. Every injury or physical skirmish left its mark on the landscape of my body.

Yet what I truly disliked, in certain gloomy moments and not always consciously, was my skin color *itself,* of which all that other piffle was merely a reminder. The insidious reasons for a brown girl's self-loathing won't be surprising to any woman of color. I cannot rightly compare my own struggles to those of another minority, as each ethnicity comes with its own baggage and the South Asian experience is just one variation on the experience of dark-skinned people everywhere. As parents and grandparents often do in Asian countries, my extended family urged me to avoid the sun, not out of fear that heatstroke would sicken me or that UV rays would lead to cancer, but more, I think, out of fear that my skin would darken to the shade of an Untouchable, a person from the lowest caste in Indian society, someone who toils in the fields. The judgments implicit in these exhortations—and what they mean about your worth— might not dawn on you while you're playing cricket in the sand. What's at stake might not dawn on you while, as a girl, you clutch fast to yourself your blonde-haired, blue-eyed doll named Helen. But all along, the message that lighter skin is equivalent to a more attractive, worthier self is getting beamed deep into your subconscious. Western ideals of beauty do not stop at ocean shores. They pervade the world and mingle with those of your own country to create mutant, unachievable standards. The prizing of lighter skin did not reach our shores with colonialism, either, for there is much reference to the virtues of fair skin in ancient Indian texts. The logic of the-lighter-the-better comforts you until suddenly you are the darker one. Our attitudes toward skin color are manifold and nuanced and even contradictory. Kids who did not think twice about calling me "blackie" in high school were still quite capable of smearing suntan oil on themselves and lying out for incessant hours to get a tan.

When I came to the U.S., of course, I saw people in many shades. It was strange and wonderful to see Chinese and Caucasian and Dominican people all riding the same subway. I was fascinated by all the different types of people, not only by their skin colors and hair textures but also by the many different ways in which they dressed and expressed themselves. It was exciting to be a kid in New York City. Over time, I started to realize, however, that certain groups of people were viewed differently than others. It was confusing. The discrimination and racism faced by African Americans was obvious to me, even as a young child. I wasn't black, but my own brown skin seemed to come with stories I hadn't written myself. During the next decade and a half, I'd gradually learn that to many Americans, my skin color signaled third-world slums as seen in Indiana Jones movies, malaria, hot curry and "stinky" food, and strange bright clothing—a caricature of India and Indians. I began to change into a person who contained two people within herself: a girl proud of and connected to her culture and native country, and one who wished she just looked like her old doll, Helen. By high school, when fitting in seems almost as important as breathing, that second girl began to take control. When I changed my name—from Padma to Angelique—for approximately four wince-worthy years, I was trying to hide from my identity. That would come later, once we had moved to California, but my divided self began to split in New York, after the second reunion with my mother.

When I returned to finish fourth grade at PS 158, I joined my mother in Manhattan at 504 East Eighty-First Street, down the street from Mr. Chip's Coffee Shop and Touch of Class cleaners, just two blocks from where we had started our life in America. I had a ball going to import stores like Azuma in the Village to decorate our new bachelorette pad—a studio apartment we divided with a yellow curtain to hide our bed. My mother's heart must have been broken and aching at her second failed marriage, but she did not stop whatever activity was in progress to show it.

My mother had a way of making every task a more elaborate happening than it needed to be. She loved the ritual of things. Far from her own culture, and ripped away time and again from her family, she ardently made every shopping trip an excursion, every grocery run a treasure hunt, every unexpected visit by a family member an impromptu dinner party. She had the charming but exhausting habit of conceiving and cooking literally a dozen different dishes for each of these visits, all out of her tiny kitchen with no window. Our friends and family took to dropping in on us without warning so as to not impose on the already tiring schedule of a single mom working by day and studying for a graduate degree by night. I don't know when Mother found the hours to do all of it, but she did, willingly, and with a smile. She relished planning a menu in bed late the night before a gathering. I thought she was talking to me, but mostly she was talking aloud to herself about what spices she would use, concocting new chutneys in her head, rehearsing new experiments using funny American ingredients like Cream of Wheat or pasta shells with South Asian spices and vegetables. She sniffed out rare Asian flora like fresh coriander and sugarcane, not at all found easily on the northeastern coast of America in the late 1970s. The experiments were always wildly pungent, and mostly all delicious.

Our neighbors, stay-at-home mothers from down the hall, often offered me bologna and cheese sandwiches with something like misty, righteous pity glimmering in their eyes.

But I loved my mother's cooking. I didn't eat ham yet or whatever that mystery meat was. And I liked watching her—not only in the kitchen. She was incredibly glamorous. Once she shed her nurse's uniform, she was liberated and instantly transformed. She got dressed to go out, spraying Norell perfume into her décolletage, trying to obscure the lingering aroma of cumin left in her cleavage from cooking my dinner. She wore heavy eye makeup with robin's egg–blue eye shadow, rouge, and bright lipstick, the whole nine yards in the brightest colors. She had taken makeup lessons from an aging, striking Swedish model who ran them out of her home. I watched *The Dukes of Hazzard* with the model's son in his bedroom while out in their living room, the women practiced on each other. I still remember the view over the city from their high-rise apartment. Our only windows looked out onto another building's wall.

I couldn't wait for her to leave after those nights of self-adornment, so I could climb onto the sink, open the medicine cabinet, and use all the tempting colors with abandon on my own face. Like a harlequin at the circus, I drew big, deep semicircles for eyebrows, coloring under them with the blue eye shadow. I often fell asleep like that, streaking the sheets with her grease paint. She never got mad, though, not once.

My mother even paid me to do chores and groom her. I got five dollars for plucking her eyebrows, a raise from my starting pay of three dollars, and I got a buck for vacuuming, since our place was quite small. I would buy vegetables at Finest grocery store on York on my way home from school, and I could make an extra couple of bucks if I washed the produce and broke off the ends of beans. I don't know how she afforded to live in the city on her nurse's salary and do all the things we miraculously did.

After a year in our cozy little studio, when my mom finally disentangled herself legally from V., we moved to California. Another new beginning. My mother tried to convince me I'd be happier in our new apartment, where, for the first time in my life, I would have my own room. I would even have my own shelf in the kitchen for my beloved Pringles. I was angry at her for moving us out of New York, however, and never really forgave her until I was well into my twenties, shelf of Pringles notwithstanding. My mother must have been tired. Her feet and heart must have ached from the tap dancing and rebuilding and continual starting over. She hated the New York winters. A little girl is a wonderful source of joy and love, and even comfort, to any mother. But I look back now and realize how lonely she must have been. How alone without any support, or anyone to talk to, in bed or elsewhere, other than me. We were extremely close, but as a child I had no sense of what she might have needed as an adult.

When we first arrived, we spent the summer in the city of Orange, near Disneyland, on the pullout couch in my uncle Bharat's family room. After that we moved to a two-bedroom rental in Arcadia, about fifteen miles northeast of L.A. Every day, my mom rode the bus for twenty minutes from Arcadia to City of Hope, the hospital where she worked. She hadn't yet learned to drive.

While the apartment itself felt almost palatial compared with our studio on the Upper East Side, I was put off by the calm and quiet of my new home. I had always lived in a metropolis. First it was Delhi, then Chennai, then New York. Now I felt burdened by the lack of bustle, the empty sidewalks, and the looming San Gabriel Mountains. I missed Gracie Mansion and the East River, which to me at the time had the romance of the Seine. In New York, I had had a measure of real independence. If I was hungry, I could stroll down the block and get a bagel and cream cheese at the Jewish deli. I could grab an after-school slice and a soda (for one dollar!) at the pizzeria. I could roller-skate, alone, the eleven blocks south to Sloan Kettering and meet my mother at work. I felt like a *person*, albeit a small one. In Arcadia, however, I felt like a kid. I had to rely on my mom for almost everything.

And Arcadia was strange and foreign to me in another, equally isolating way: it was populated mostly by white people and a small smattering of Asians—Koreans, Chinese, and Filipinos. Other than my mother and my reflection in the mirror, I effectively saw just one other Indian: my uncle. He was married to my aunt Trudy, a Swiss woman, so their kids, Sheila and Ashok, were half Indian, half Swiss ethnically, but were otherwise pretty much brown-skinned American kids from Orange County, California. They did not identify with many things in Indian culture and only went to India once every few years. But because they were used to frequent visits from strange relatives of their father's from back home, they were incredibly nice and welcoming. My cousin Ashok was a year older than me, and his sister, Sheila, six years younger. But the three of us were close and played well together. At some point, my mother befriended a Gujarati couple, the Mishras. Pratima Mishra was an expert at assimilating non-Indian ingredients into her cooking. Often, she would deep-fry whatever she found (flour tortillas cut into triangles, say) and serve it with chutney.

India, of course, was a sea of brown faces. And in New York, Indians had been everywhere, from the subcontinenters who colonized our Elmhurst apartment building, to the cab drivers who knew the quickest way to get anywhere in the city, to the doctors who worked with my mom at Sloan Kettering, to the hot dog vendors who had sold us our hot-dog-less dogs. In New York I even heard many Indian languages spoken, including Tamil. I never felt like an outsider. Or at least when I did, I knew I was in the company of many, many other outsiders. On the walk to school, whether it was in Elmhurst or on York Avenue in Manhattan, I'd pass Filipinos and Peruvians, Barbadians and Chinese, Puerto Ricans and African Americans and Middle Easterners. Even some of the white faces I saw were minorities, I learned, because they were Polish or had menorahs instead of Christmas trees. We were different from one another—we spoke different languages, ate different foods, went home to see our families in different far-flung countries—but we were alike in our differences. In that respect, New York City didn't feel that much different from India. Just as Chennai and Delhi included people from all over India with different languages, religions, and cultures, so, too, did New York, where everyone seemed united by place and shared purpose, different from one another but part of a larger sameness.

California, and especially the greater Los Angeles area, is incredibly diverse, but the vast sprawl meant that the great pockets of Mexican and Chinese and African American inhabitants, at least from my vantage point, stayed separate. In high school, I observed this in microcosm. The Filipinos hung out together. So did the Mexicans. At school, kids didn't know what to make of me. They were confused that I didn't speak Spanish. "But you look Mexican," they'd say. The types of insults and treatment I got used to in elementary school came fast and furious here, too, though they were less creative than "Black Giraffe." I was taller and ganglier than most kids in my fifth-grade class. At age ten, being tall seemed intentional, like an affront. You could almost see the contempt on the other kids' faces. *Who does she think she is, taking up all that space?* My vocabulary—nothing special, but distasteful to those who felt that trying at school was an offense almost as grave as being tall—led the kids to call me "Dictionary" behind my back. Becky liked to yank my hair from behind me in English class. David stuck to giving me flat tires by stepping on my heels as we walked to class, making me struggle to get my shoes back on, and frequently called me the N-word in my sixth-grade class. I got egged in seventh grade on the last day of school. I was punched by a girl in the face; then an egg was smashed on top of my head. I remember banging on Mr. Piela's classroom door, dripping with yolk and gooey ooze all in my hair, pleading for him to let me in. I was bullied and humiliated and relieved that school was over and we were moving. We only lived a couple of years in the mostly white enclave of Arcadia, then moved to a more working-class neighborhood in another part of the Valley where my mom and her boyfriend could afford to buy a house. In eighth grade at Sierra Vista Junior High, in La Puente, I became perhaps the world's least popular cheerleader. I suspect that the teachers, who liked me because I worked hard, ensured that I made the squad. The rest of the girls definitely did not approve. For the first time in my life, even after a childhood spent shuttling between New York and India, I felt foreign. I felt like I didn't belong.

To make matters worse, this was around the time I met Peter. We had only been in Los Angeles for two years. I was still in sixth grade, living in our apartment in Arcadia, when I came out of my room one morning to the sight of a man snoring loudly on the divan in a big, dark heap. He had greasy hair and skin the color of mahogany leather. A beer belly leaked out of the space between his tattered T-shirt and paint-speckled jeans. I was scared of this man, of his big, knotty, callused hands, of his smell, sour like old beer and tobacco. Two years later, he would become my stepfather.

"Mom!" I yelled. "Who is this man?"

She explained that she had hired him, a friend of a friend, to build us a stereo cabinet. For some reason, he had decided to show up at 6:00 a.m. on a Saturday, too early for hammering. She told him so and suggested he lie down for a while. When the sleeping giant awoke, he clomped around in his work boots and spoke to my mother in bass, tortured Hindi. My preteen self immediately hated him.

Born and raised in Fiji, Peter descended from generations of lower-caste Indians whom the British shipped as indentured laborers to colonies like Fiji and Guyana with the promise of a better life. He immigrated to California directly from Fiji, working first as a gardener. Historically, the Indian migrants to Fiji had a combative relationship with Fiji's indigenous peoples. Afraid of losing their culture to that of their adoptive home, they clung to it. While India moved forward, the insularity of these transplants kept them culturally frozen in time. Gender roles were sharply defined. Women had little say; they belonged at home. Punishment of children was always corporal. Girls were to be married off, fraternizing with the opposite sex was forbidden.

In part because of his size but mainly because of what I saw as his crude, beast-like ignorance, I referred to Peter when speaking to my mom in private as "the Incredible Hulk." I was too young to understand how he went from cabinet builder to main squeeze. All I knew was that I didn't like him. I didn't like his big belt buckle, his stench, his coarse way. I didn't like his Hindi, which bore a thick island drawl—ugly, I thought then.

I wanted my mom to be with someone more cultured. Not this man who had never visited India, this farmer with an eighth-grade education, this brute who would unleash strings of curses from the front door when an unsuspecting boy classmate dared to walk me home and set foot on Peter's lawn. How could my mom, who in New York had stretched her income to take me to movies and museums and Broadway shows, who held a master's degree in public health, date this man so far beneath her? I felt entitled to judge her choice of companion. Her choice of companion drastically affected my daily home life, and suddenly our home became known at my high school as the house with the irascible, ill-tempered stepdad. Over time he would repeatedly go back to school to study for various trade licenses, like plumbing, contracting, and even real estate. Many years after his intrusion into my life, this giant and I would bond deeply through the love we shared for my daughter and my mother—this ogre turned out to be more Shrek than Grendel. Now he is my daughter's closest grandparent, playing physically with her and spoiling her in a way no one else can.

Through the decades, I've thought hard about the reasons behind the virulence of my initial reaction to Peter. There was, of course, his interruption of the intimacy my mother and I shared. I didn't like his intrusion into our life. For years, it had been just the two of us against the world. There was also my history with wannabe fathers: first my birth father's abandonment of me, and the second divorce because V. had not believed us. They had hurt me and they had hurt my mother. I felt I had to protect us both. And finally, there was a more subtle reason: I had begun to internalize the judgment I felt for being Indian, for being dark-skinned, for being from a poor, strange country. Then Peter came along and made manifest everything I hated about who people thought I was. I changed my name just as my mother and Peter were getting close.

My new name came from my mother's friend, a fellow nurse at City of Hope named Angie. I looked forward to the days when she'd come over. A short, round Colombian woman, she had a mane of lush dark-brown blow-dried locks, feathered to perfection like Jaclyn Smith's on *Charlie's Angels*. Her skin glowed, even though I couldn't detect any makeup on her face, except for approximately six coats of mascara on her spidery lashes. I had never seen someone so beautiful. She showed up in her all-white nurse's outfit (dress, stockings, shoes) straight from work with my mom. She and my mom would sit at our coffee table, my mom with her lentils and rice and Angie with a Styrofoam box of takeout. I'm still not sure why Angie never ate my mother's food. She may have felt about it the way I felt about eating meat. Maybe she felt bad straining my mother's resources.

I'd corner Angie on the couch and interrogate her. How come your hair is so bouncy? What shampoo do you use? Do you sleep with curlers, like Alice from *The Brady Bunch*? How did you get your eyelashes to look so beautiful? Her answer to that last question I still remember: Apply coat after coat of mascara, letting each dry before adding the next. And, she said, warning me not to, she separated them with the tip of a safety pin. She answered each question with evident pleasure. I watched her around others and she had the same sunny, soothing way with them. I wished to be like Angie and have the effect on people that she did. I also knew that she lived with her mother, who was sick with cancer. Angie would phone her and speak in the most melodic Spanish. Her voice as she spoke to her mother reminded me of Elena, my old Peruvian babysitter in Elmhurst. Elena never became flustered, even with half a dozen other people's kids buzzing around her and her husband coming home for supper soon. She catered to everyone and made you feel that even the most annoying, chaotic scene was just fine, just part of a normal day. I loved her ability to make everything all right with calm.

One day in late August, right before we moved from Arcadia to the house in La Puente, Angie asked me if I was excited to go to my new junior high school. I said no. I had gone to two different schools already since we had moved to L.A., and what I dreaded most was having to repeat my name over and over again to a whole new batch of people. I dreaded roll call, when the teacher would come to my name on the attendance sheet— the long pause, the stuttering and stumbling.

It hurt even more because part of me liked my name. My given name was Padma Parvati Vaidyanathan. In modern Tamilian tradition, your father's first name becomes your last name until you marry, when it surrenders to your husband's. When my mother married, she became Vijayalakshmi Vaidyanathan. After her divorce, she dropped her husband's name. Instead of reverting to her father's name, she split her first name in two and Lakshmi became her and my last name. It was Rajima's second name too, after all. My mother's decision was both a form of feminist defiance and a matter of practicality. The traditional culture of Kerala, where our family is from, is indeed matrilineal, so the split felt like honoring her roots. It was also a matter of pride: she refused to be tagged by men. She would no longer be defined in those terms, as a daughter or a wife. I was proud to have a name that reflected her courage. As a practical matter, having more digestible names would help our transition from India to America.

Yet, reflected in the mirror of others' reactions, my name came to seem distorted, strange, and a little icky. As icky in their eyes as what my mom would sometimes pack for me for lunch. I'll never forget the grimaces at the lunch table from friends and acquaintances who, having unwrapped their PB&Js, would spot (and smell) the contents of my square Tupperware container. My rice and curry, which I loved and which I admit was, like most Indian food, fragrant (to put it generously), inspired many an "Ew, what is *that*?"

At the time, Indian culture had none of the cachet it would acquire decades later and now possesses. By 1984, my native country had had only one major moment in popular American culture, inspired by rock stars. The Beatles had gone to India in 1968 to meditate at an ashram in the city of Rishikesh. The press covered the visit with such wonderment that soon afterward, Westerners were toting books of Indian lore and spirituality, and dorms filled with the scent of *nag champa* incense and patchouli oil. Life became all peace and love and maharishi. More than thirty years later, another rock star, Madonna, would take up yoga and former aerobics instructors everywhere would discover the glories of *pincha mayurasana* and *halsana* poses. After college, when I went to yoga classes in L.A., I would giggle so hard at the Valley-accented approximations of *chataranga* that I could barely hold my downward-facing dog. But that wouldn't happen for another ten years or so.

At the time I became Angelique, India—for most Americans I encountered—connoted smelly, poor, and weird. I felt both American and Indian. But I had to pick a side, and I decided I'd choose the least conspicuous one. I wanted to fade in, not stand out. A new school meant another round of hazing, but as I realized after my conversation with Angie, it also presented an opportunity for reinvention. And while I couldn't change the way I looked, I could change my name.

Now all I needed was the right one. I wanted something approachable, something that didn't sound foreign, that would make no waves. I thought of Angie, the way I felt when I heard my mom say her name. I liked that name. Not so long ago, there had been a sitcom of the same name. That proved to me that most Americans were familiar with the name Angie. I told my mom of my plan. I suspect she was heartbroken, even though she never showed it. In fact, she encouraged me to find a name with which I felt more at ease, one that "fit" better. I told her my choice, and she suggested that I should ask Angie. So the next time they came home together from work, I gushed that I had always loved her and her name and I would like to use it as my own in my new school and would that be okay?

Angie listened patiently. I made sure to mention that even Peter had changed *his* name from Anand when he first arrived from Fiji. When I was done presenting my case, Angie told me she thought my name was very special. She looked to my mother and asked whether she was all right with the change. My mother set Angie's hot tea on a coaster on the coffee table and assured her that she wouldn't stand in my way if that was what I wanted. Angie met my mother's eyes, as if trying to divine the role my mother expected her to play. Eventually, graciously, she assented. She was flattered, she said.

The first day of each new semester, I'd eagerly wait as the teacher took attendance, ready for her to reach the last names beginning with L. I could sense the moment when she reached my name. I could spot the beginning of the furrowed brow that preceded the stutter, "P-P-Pad . . ." And I spoke up immediately. "Here!" I'd say. "Call me Angie." I wasn't the only one with a new name. Hae Sun became Susie. Marisol became Lisa. I'm pretty sure my friend Lynn was not a true Lynn. I never thought to ask.

I was Angie for a year. As the shock of yet another new school wore off, I drifted back toward the exotic. I then elongated and embellished the name to Angelique the year after. I suppose I wanted to be noticed, just not for the reasons I was noticed as Padma. But of course my skin color and the other markers of my ethnicity—my dark eyes and fine, straight black hair—were immutable.

So all through eighth grade I was Angie, and for the entirety of high school, my friends and teachers called me Angelique. My mother feigned indifference, a sort of neutral support. If asked by other relatives for her opinion, she would simply say, "Well, I named her Padma, but if she doesn't like it, what can I do? Let her be called what she wants." She even went so far as to call me Angelique when speaking to me around my friends, with only the faintest whiff of resignation. I'm sure she noticed that I never ate at the table and stayed mostly in my room. At the time my household environment was stressful, to say the least, and I wasn't comfortable in my own home. I felt it wasn't fair that I had no control over whom I lived with. My mother knew me well. I would have balked at any serious opposition to my name change. It was one of the few things I had control over, after all.

My mother also knew I sneaked out or was picked up down the street by male friends to get around the ogre guarding our threshold.

Two years after I spotted him on the couch, Peter and my mother decided to move in together to the working-class neighborhood of La Puente, a pimple on the map between Hollywood and Disneyland. In 1984 they bought the low-slung house where they still live today. I spent most of my time locked inside my bedroom, lying on my bed, trying to lose myself in *The Outsiders*. I spent no time in my mom's bedroom, because it was Peter's room, too. The third bedroom was officially a guest room but functioned as a dumping ground for my hoarder of a mother's excess stuff. Today this room is no different, taken up by stacks of boxes, old clothing, shoes, Christmas ornaments, glue sticks, and photos of me, from ancient modeling shots to a framed one of me in cap and gown and *bindi,* my mom in a sari, beaming.

Peter created a lush garden with trees bearing kumquats, tangerines, and curry leaves, and one with roses in front of the house, for my mother. Our neighbor had a pomegranate tree that hung over the fence in our backyard. I'd wait for the pomegranates to fall before cracking them open, prying out the seeds, and dousing them with lemon and salt—*chaatpati* in a bowl. Peter tended the garden, shuffling between trees with his farmer's gait, bowlegged from the car accident we suffered in 1985 and slightly pigeon-toed. My contempt for Peter endured, and not without reason. A window next to my bed looked out onto the backyard. On certain days, I looked up from the pages of my book after hearing insistent clucking followed by a desperate squawk. I didn't have to look outside to know what it was. Peter was using his giant hands to slaughter a chicken. It would come to be a familiar sound.

The Silence of the Chickens happened every few weeks. He would chop their heads off with one swoop, dunk the still-screaming birds into a barrel of boiling water, pluck them, and use the same cleaver to hack them into indecipherable pieces. He and an enlisted friend from back home slaughtered about a dozen at a time. They divided the kill between the two of them. What my parents didn't freeze for a later date, he'd make pungent chicken curry with. The curry, as I remember it, was made from tons of garlic, onion, oil, and a coarse, stinky spice mixture. The smell was nothing like the delicate aroma of South Indian food. When it finished stewing, a slick yellow-tinged soot clung to the pot. I mostly succeeded in avoiding Peter, but occasionally we'd cross paths and I'd watch out of the corner of my eye as he ate a bowl filled with curry and a giant wedge of rice—not basmati rice but some inferior *poni* grain, microwaved. He hunched over the bowl, his left arm hugging it and his right hand dragging a cluster of stale rice through the sludge. Even from the other room, I could hear him sucking on the bones and snapping them with his teeth to get at the marrow.

He complained that the grocery store chicken had no flavor. Today I understand that he was right about that and that his way was actually much less cruel than factory farming, which produces meat sanitized of its origins by customers' remove from the gruesome particulars. But an avian bloodbath was not a convincing argument against factory farming to a teenage girl. I had been slowly incorporating meat into my Brahmin diet for a couple of years now. I was not exactly a vegetarian but still very squeamish about eating things that actually tasted and looked like meat. Peter's occasionally murderous activities meant that even the backyard was a place I didn't feel comfortable. I could no longer tell if a red splotch on the ground originated from a squashed pomegranate seed or a doomed chicken. Spotting a stray feather would send me into hysterics. I resented my mother for allowing the slaughter, though I suppose she deserves credit for drawing the line at lamb. I knew he'd lost that battle the first day I saw him walk in with a large black Hefty bag filled with parts that he'd unload into the freezer. I knew what the heavy, still-warm contents were. By that time, I was no longer a vegetarian and had no moral objection to eating meat. Peter and his relatives were Hindus, too, but not Brahmins, of course. They ate all meat except beef and pork. So he had the same reaction when I brought home a burger or cooked bacon on a Saturday morning. I was accustomed to religion restricting diet. Still, I couldn't understand (or refused to consider) why he would eat lamb and chicken but not beef or pork. He was a hypocrite, I decided. And disgusting.

The days of my mom and I working as a team in the kitchen were over. Now she would come home from work, cook dinner, and leave it on the stove. I'd emerge from my bedroom only to make myself a plate, then go straight back to my room and shut the door. I was horrible to Peter. When he spoke to me in Hindi, I'd snap, "I can't understand you, what language is that?" I'd speak to my mom almost exclusively in Tamil, which I knew he couldn't understand. He'd sigh and say, *"Mabitiya, mabitiya"* ("Mother-daughter, mother-daughter"), as if to say that we were in a club he wasn't part of. *Yep, pretty much,* I thought.

Blinded by my disapproval and adolescent certainty, I couldn't see Peter's struggle. If I had been watching, I would have seen him try hard to reconcile his old ways with his new family. He loved my mother, I could see that, and he was trying to show affection for me. He did this the only way he knew how, through fierce protection. Like when senior prom rolled around. I had won a free limo ride in a lunchtime raffle, but I had no date and insufficient courage to go with just my girlfriends. A week or so before the big dance, a junior boy came up to me. "I heard you don't have a date to prom," he said, before adding, "and that you won the limo." Talk about sweeping a girl off her feet. "I'll go with you," I said. "Just don't touch me above the knees or below the neck." Peter, as I expected, refused to be in the house when the boy arrived. But I later found out that he paid for a couple extra hours of limo time. In retrospect, I think his outbursts had an ostentatious quality. He had a very big temper and often got into fights at the local bar, the ironically named Hi Brow Lounge, where the area painters, plumbers, and electricians drank. He became unreasonable when he drank, and our linen closet for years had a different-colored piece of wood on one of the doors from when he kicked a hole through it during one of his outbursts. If an unwitting boy stopped to speak to me on my front lawn after school, in broad daylight, he would come out of the garage where he kept his tools, swinging a wrench and spurting obscenities. I could never do group projects with male students, as they weren't allowed in my home. We did have many Mexican and Filipino kids at my high school whose parents had similarly conservative attitudes, but none as backward as his. He did not tolerate any socialization between the sexes. And no one was as scary as he was. He had Fijian friends in the neighborhood; perhaps he wanted to prove his conservative bona fides. They all had clung to ancient Indian customs that were archaic even when compared with those of my South Indian grandfather, whose private tutorial business out of our home in Chennai frequently had students of both sexes studying together and milling around the house. In Peter's community, quite literally everyone had arranged marriages; no one was even allowed a say in the matter. Even my mother's upbringing a generation earlier in India had been more liberal than what Peter allowed in our shared home.

My mother tried to mediate between us, to no avail. It got so bad that once, near the end of my sophomore year, Peter actually tried to run me over with his work truck. Or at least to scare me pretty bad. My mom had to go to a nurses' conference in Baltimore, and by then I had an after-school job at Robinson's department store. I was late to work and a friend offered me a ride. I was very nervous that Peter would come home, since his schedule was erratic, depending on whatever jobs he had on any given day. When D. pulled up into my driveway in his pickup truck, I dashed out to get into the passenger seat. D., trying to be a gentleman, got out of the car to let me into my side. I got in as fast as I could. D. walked around to get back into the car as Peter drove up.

I begged D. to hurry but the next thing I knew, we were being rear-ended by Peter's work truck. D., of course, was shocked and stunned. My stepdad yelled curse words from behind the wheel as he repeatedly backed up and then rear-ended us several times really hard. I begged D. to stay in the vehicle, even though with every bang the whole truck shook forward. Peter was yelling for us to "get the fuck out of" his driveway but somewhere in his blinding rage he must have realized we could not do this if he was behind us. Peter finally backed up one last time and parked his vehicle on the street. He got out and kicked and dented the side of poor D.'s white Toyota pickup. D., not a small guy himself, was pretty cool about the whole thing. He drove me to the Puente Hills Mall as I sobbed next to him.

When I finished work, I decided I had had enough. I went to a friend's home and called my mother at her Maryland hotel. I told her what had happened and that I refused to go back into that crazy house. I stayed with my friend until my mother came home. I refused to live there any longer and told her if she wanted to stay she could. Needless to say, the dynamic between Peter and me caused severe strain on my relationship with my mother, which until Peter came along had pretty much been idyllic. She and I moved into a rental nearby with a colleague of hers from the hospital shortly before my junior year in high school. I was baffled by my mother's love for Peter. She had always raised me in an open and liberal way. Now we were forced to live according to his ignorant standards of what was appropriate.

But we were not totally disconnected from him. I knew my mom still saw him on the sly. And when I turned sixteen at the end of that summer, he helped me to buy a car, strangely from a senior male student, coming with me to check it out and giving me the three hundred dollars as a gift for my birthday to buy it. He must have been very conflicted, trying to reconcile his ways with ours and trying to control his temper, with little success.

Peter got the brunt of my teenage hate and myopia. The rest went to my mother. I was a decent kid, too much of a goody-goody for drinking or drugs—my only form of rebellion was the menthol cigarettes, long and gruesome, that I hid in the glove box of my copper-brown Ford Pinto. I was not, however, immune to impressive feats of self-absorption. At the time, I didn't see my mother for the person she was beyond her motherly duties. For instance, she had a great capacity for nurturing. Years before she and I moved out of the house we shared with Peter, I understood this only from the little things she did for me. In the winter, before each day of school, my mom would put my jeans in the dryer so I could have the pleasure of slipping on heated pants. Late at night, I'd call out and she'd bring me a glass of milk, even though I was far too old to be scared of the dark and even closer than she was to the kitchen. Through the years, hospitalizations, and surgeries to come, she'd drop everything to fly to my side and care for me. I took this as a given, as what any mother would do for her daughter. But as an adult I came to understand that this was who she was as a person, not just as a mother. It was so much a part of her that she chose a career devoted to the service of others.

When the AIDS epidemic began, she left City of Hope to become a hospice nurse. I remember coming home one Friday during freshman year to find blueberries in the fridge. Before I could eat them by the handful, she warned me to leave them alone. I begged and pleaded, to no avail. They were for Robert. Robert had been one of her patients for six months. She adored him. He had advanced AIDS and was feeling particularly bad of late. Recently he had shared with my mother fond memories of going blueberry picking as a child. She thought that bringing him this basket of berries when she returned to work on Monday might give him some small measure of joy.

But when I came home from school that Monday, my mother said I could eat the berries. I didn't stop to think what this might mean. My concerns were fully contained in the small, self-absorbed box of adolescence. I couldn't imagine the world in which her patients existed. So I didn't try to. I happily grabbed the container from the fridge and popped handfuls of berries into my mouth as I did my homework. Robert had died, of course, and when I found out, I didn't feel sadness for him, his family, or even my mother. All I felt was profound guilt for the pleasure I took in eating those berries.

The summer before senior year, I left our little rental and went to India for three months, as I always did, and halfway through, my mother showed up with Peter in tow, hand in hand as if there had never been a separation. I was livid and determined to get out of that house, and college seemed to be a legitimate escape route.

I didn't go back to calling myself Padma until applying to college. I saw a poster for Clark University in faraway Worcester, Massachusetts, at a college fair. The poster had a picture of a half-open pea pod with different-colored peas nestled into it. "Categorizing people isn't something you can do here," read the caption. That was the college for me. Not only was it clear on the other side of the country, away from Peter, away from that house and everything else I had always hated about my home life, but it seemed to be telling me that on its campus I could be myself. I had also just come back from India and was bolstered by a fresh reminder of myself at home there. I began to see that changing my name was futile. A name is a marker of identity, but there are markers we cannot change, like the color of our bodies.

As a model, through my failures and successes, I felt conflicted. I liked who I was, but I also wished I could be a more salable color, a better commodity, a toothpaste-commercial-worthy girl. It took years for this internalized self-loathing to fade.

Still, the tension remains. It always will. When I look at my daughter, with her green eyes and light skin but with my bone structure, I see the strange reflection of the "me" I had long wanted to be. The funny thing is, when she looks back at me, she covets all the features I once wanted gone. She begs me to straighten her light, ringletted hair. She wishes she had brown eyes. She yearns for the dark shade of my skin and fights with those in her class who tell her she doesn't look Indian. "Don't worry, *kanna*, you're brown on the inside," I joke to her.

chapter 6

I had no intention of being a TV host when I attended Clark, where I majored in theater arts and minored in American literature.

By my senior year, I was bored of campus life. The surrounding city of Worcester (pronounced, with a thud, as "Wooster") wasn't exactly a hub of culture and opportunity. So I wiggled my way last minute into a spring-semester-long study-abroad program in Madrid for my last months of college life. I spoke no Spanish. My first choice was Paris, though I didn't speak French, either, but our university's French program was in Dijon. Since I was a city girl, I opted for the metropolis of tapas and flamenco.

Between classes, I'd walk the city. With its squares and grand buildings, Madrid looked the way I had imagined Paris would. I was excited to be in Europe. I experienced no culture shock, even though it was my first time there. Perhaps all that shuttling I had done between India and America had helped me become a curious and unencumbered traveler. By the fall of my senior year, I had grown out of Clark, and Worcester was starting to look as small as La Puente had four years earlier. I stayed with a family in the Argüelles neighborhood in Madrid. The mother of the family I lived with came home every day to cook elaborate meals for lunch. I couldn't believe she left work just to make freshly breaded cutlets of veal or pounded chicken with potatoes and salad for the family, only to then take the subway back to work without observing the siesta, except for a brief time she lay on the couch with her legs up as she smoked her black Ducados cigarettes. I discovered that after the post-lunch siesta came a magic time for starving students. With dinner an eternity away at nine thirty, you could kill a few hours nursing a small beer at a bar and eating your fill in free tapas, perhaps salt cod on toast, *papas bravas* (fried potatoes topped with a thick, pimentón-spiked sauce), or a little dish of olives.

I knew only one person in Madrid: Santiago Molina, a friend from Clark who had graduated a year before me. Santiago chivalrously took care of me in Madrid. A platonic friend, sweet as can be, he picked me up at the airport when I arrived, bought me drinks when we went out, and showed me around the city. I was eager for culture, though far from cultured myself. He took me to the Prado—which I mistakenly called the Prada, wondering to myself why an Italian design house would own a Spanish art museum—where I spent hours lingering in front of works by Goya, Velázquez, Bosch, and Rubens.

A couple of weeks after I got to Madrid, Santiago took me to a bar called Zarabanda, where we met up with a friend of his, a tall, beautiful man named Fernando. He worked as a booker at a modeling agency called (I kid you not) Jet Set, and Santiago joked that I could model for him. I'll never forget what Fernando did in response. He took a step toward me, so his face was inches from mine. As I looked into his eyes, the bluest I've ever seen, he reached out his big hands and took my face in them. I might have swooned if he weren't as gay as he was gorgeous. His fingers fondled my jaw and cheekbones, as if he were inspecting the wrapper of a Mars bar in order to tell whether the candy inside had melted. "Maybe," he said. "She has good bones."

The next day, Santiago suggested we visit Fernando at his office. "You just want to meet models," I replied. "Yeah, so what," he said, smiling mischievously. Then he reminded me of my dire financial situation. I would soon graduate with a theater degree and a mountain of student loan debt. Extra pocket money couldn't hurt. Money aside, I was secretly excited. Like many girls, I had a serious fashion magazine habit. I knew all about designers like Chanel and Yves Saint Laurent, Armani and the rest. I envied the models pictured in those pages—Christy, Linda, Cindy—but I knew I wasn't model material.

Sure, I thought I looked very cool at the time in my pilly oversized sweater, leggings, and knee-high fake leather boots. I wouldn't be surprised if the sweater had shoulder pads. I understood that I was cute enough to flirt my way into a nightclub, but that was about as far as my looks could get me. The women in fashion magazines weren't just a different degree of pretty from me. They were a different kind, like a different race born with glossy long limbs and perfect skin and white teeth. Speaking of race, modeling seemed to me the domain of white girls. I had yet to see Yasmeen Ghauri, a stunning half-Pakistani, half-German model, grace the cover of *Cosmo* in pink satin. Santiago had to drag me to the agency. But a part of me, at least, was happy to be dragged.

We met Fernando at Jet Set. Whatever I was wearing that day—most likely another big-sweater-over-leggings combo—I was not dressed like a girl who was about to have a modeling audition. He led us to a room dominated by a sort of jerry-rigged runway, where Josette Naimas, the owner of the agency, soon joined us. Josette was Brazilian, her skin approximately the same color as mine. She looked elegant in her burgundy cashmere sweater and suede pants, with her dark coiffed hair, like a longer version of Anne Bancroft's in *The Graduate*, not a strand out of place. She asked me to step up on the platform. This, I learned, was where she taught models how to walk.

She and a female booker named Peppa, who would later become a good friend, asked me to walk across the platform. *Ooookay*, I thought, as I put one foot in front of the other, trying my best to walk normally, which felt difficult now that I was being observed. After that, Josette began to inspect me. She unfurled a tape measure and wrapped it around my waist and bust. She measured my height. I knew very well how tall I was. I had reached five-foot-nine at age thirteen. I'd often taken flak for my height. My old elementary school nickname "Black Giraffe" echoed in my head. My height and long neck earned the noun. The adjective speaks, rather sadly, for itself. Later, I was called "Skeletor," after He-Man's nemesis, whom I suppose I resembled because I was naturally gaunt. By the time I was old enough to be shy around boys, I had been ridiculed for my gangliness long enough that I developed a hunch to conceal my true height. Yet in that moment, for Josette, I straightened my back to look as tall as I could. Now she was telling me I was barely tall enough. My ambivalence about this strange audition gave way to anger. Even though Josette was kind, I hated Santiago for taking me there. I felt I was being forced to participate in a contest I was ill prepared for. It was like being entered into the French Open without ever training beyond playing casual social tennis. I was pretty enough and just beginning to feel confident, and now I was being scrutinized against impossibly high standards without ever wanting to put myself up for it.

My audition was nearly over when Josette interrupted her inspection to answer a call. She hung up and engaged in a back-and-forth in rapid Spanish with Santiago. They were both looking at me. He beamed: "We're going to *Elle* magazine!" Turned out Spanish *Elle* needed an exotic girl to be a fitting model. Fitting models are the lowest rung on the modeling ladder. They're essentially live mannequins that editors dress in various outfits, testing the looks before the shoot with the real model—in this case, almost certainly a girl with my dark skin tone. I couldn't believe it. My anger quickly turned to exhilaration. I didn't care if I was walking a runway or the floor of a restaurant carrying a tray of drinks. I had a job! But now that I did, I knew that I had to come clean. My stomach knotted and my heart sank.

"Wait!" I said, as they started making arrangements to send me to *Elle*'s offices. Before Josette and Fernando and everyone else embarrassed themselves by submitting me to *Elle*, they had to know that I was a lemon—a decent-looking car with a bum transmission. "I have a scar," I announced. No one was listening. "A very big scar," I boomed. I pulled up the sleeve of my turtleneck and revealed the ropy line of swollen tissue, seven inches long and as thick as a garter snake, on my right arm.

The accident happened on a Sunday afternoon filled with sunshine. I was fourteen years old, driving home with my mom and Peter from a Hindu temple in Malibu. We had an old Mercury sedan, the kind with bench seats in front and back. I was sitting up front, between Peter and my mom, because I had been severely ill and hospitalized, only to be discharged two days earlier. The traffic on the 101 freeway was quite heavy for a Sunday but, oddly, moving at a very fast speed nonetheless. I remember thinking how strange that was. Then there was a loud bang, and I looked out the windshield and saw nothing but the prettiest blue sky. I thought I was dreaming, because I'd been nodding off, but then I realized we were part of that sky. Our red Ford Mercury was airborne. Arcing through the air in that car felt like an exhilarating hallucination, an unbelievable ride that oddly remains one of the most beautiful images in my memory.

We were airborne for what seemed like a very long time, flying off the freeway, then forty feet down the embankment. I remember watching the car door swing open and shut on one of Peter's legs as we flew, while he clutched the steering wheel to keep himself inside. There was a tremendous bang as we hit a tree, then a crash as the tree fell on the car, crushing the roof and pinning the three of us against the seat—our strange family suddenly forced together and confronted with more than just dysfunction. My right arm, which I had thrown across my mother's chest, perhaps in a vain effort to protect her, took the brunt of the impact from the roof. Yet this impact was so strong that after crushing my arm, it also broke her sternum, five ribs, and her arm. Things went black.

Then I remember opening my eyes in the car. Blood, glass, dirt, and leaves were everywhere. I could barely turn my head, and when I did I saw that my mother was unconscious, blood trickling from her mouth. Peter was muttering, confused. "Where are we?" he asked. "What's going on?" I would remain conscious, covered in glass, for the hour and a half it took for the paramedics and firefighters to get through the traffic and hike from the road down the embankment. My body went into shock, shivering uncontrollably, but I felt no pain. They used the Jaws of Life to open the car roof like a tin of sardines. A helicopter landed in the middle of the freeway to take my parents away to USC Medical Center. An ambulance carried me to Queen of Angels Hospital, where I finally lost consciousness without knowing whether my mother and her husband were alive.

When I woke up hours later, I had tubes coming out of several places in my body. My right arm had been shattered, my right index metacarpal severed, and my left hip fractured. Shards of glass had embedded themselves in my skin, under my nails. To this day I have a shard lingering in my right thumb. My mother and Peter, I soon found out, were alive. Peter had broken his leg in four places and his hip in two. My mother was hurt the worst. She had snapped five ribs and her sternum, as well as her left hand and right arm. She had been airlifted because the impact had squeezed her heart. Her body and her spirit have never recovered completely. She no longer drives on freeways. When I'm in town, she often chooses to sit in the backseat with my daughter, which I think makes her happy in more ways than one. When she does ride in the front seat, I can sense her anxiety. Even as I ease to a stop, I often see her hands clutch the dashboard and her foot jam an imaginary brake pedal.

After my first surgery, I was left with the scar, thin and straight, on my right arm. I was so grateful for the use of my arm that I didn't think much of it. The doctors suggested that it might even get thinner and less noticeable. Instead, over the three or so years after the accident, I developed a keloid and the scar transformed into the gnarly caterpillar that today creeps up my right arm. Perhaps I could've asked the doctor to cut on the underside of the arm instead, where the scar would have been hidden. But at the time, of course, I was in no state to make such aesthetics-based decisions.

When we got out of the hospital, we recovered at home, each of us too injured to minister to the others. We had home health nurses who looked after us. My aunt Trudy visited frequently and helped tend to us. As we healed on the outside, we all struggled inside, in our own quiet ways. My struggle was one of faith. The accident alone didn't bring this about. Just a couple of days before the crash, I had finished a long stay at City of Hope Hospital. My mother had wanted to give penance and perform a *puja* of thanks at a temple, and the nearest Hindu temple was in Malibu, fifty miles from our home.

Several weeks earlier, I'd developed Stevens-Johnson syndrome, a rare and life-threatening condition caused by an adverse reaction to medication or to a virus. Ulcers and lesions attacked and scalded my eyes, mouth, and throat. I'd first gone to a local hospital, but even the electric ice bed they put me on couldn't lower my fever. My mother slept in the hospital, slumped on a chair or in a free bed beside me—as she's done every time I've been hospitalized since, even when I've begged her to leave—while doctors tried and failed to diagnose my illness. She was fierce, my mother, and refused to accept incompetence. After days, she hired a private ambulance, unhooked my IV bag from its hook, and led me out of there with the IV still tethered to my arm. She took me to City of Hope, where she worked. The ulcers and sores rendered me essentially blind and mute for three interminable weeks. I was in terrible pain. I could not swallow my own saliva and had to sleep sitting up. At five-foot-nine, I weighed ninety-eight pounds.

From these events I took away a new suspicion of comfort and happiness, understanding they were impermanent and could be taken away at any time. My family and I were pretty secular, but I believed in God and took our Hindu rituals seriously. Exacting this kind of karma seemed cruel if there was a God. Hadn't my mom's life been hard enough? I experienced a bout of atheism. With adolescent self-importance, I wondered why God would allow all this to happen to a fourteen-year-old girl.

When I was finally able to resume my normal life, I focused on making up the months of schoolwork I'd missed while in the hospital and then recovering at home. I was out until May, and even when I went back to school, I had grueling physical therapy to reeducate my arm three times a week before school started as it was frozen and immobile at a ninety-degree angle at my side. I tried to move forward. The scar, however, was there to remind me and everyone else of what had happened. It caught everyone's eye, a ropy and gnarled raised keloid. And I could see the look of wonder and shock on other people's faces when they met me for the first time after the accident. I thought it was ugly, and it embarrassed me to no end. I became very self-conscious about it. I wore long sleeves when I could. For those times when I couldn't, I perfected a casual pose that hid the scar under my left hand and raised thumb when my arms were crossed. I had always stood out for my height and skin color. But now, all people seemed to notice was the scar.

I overheard the pity-ridden compliments. "It's such a shame," people would say. "She was so pretty. She could have modeled." Just months before the accident, when my mom was in the midst of a very eighties series of self-help seminars designed to release one's inner child, I joined her for one of these sessions. That's where we met a photographer, who asked my mother if he could take some pictures of me. Reluctantly, she agreed. A week later, she held the light reflector for him under the Santa Monica Pier. The photos were beautiful; even the brooding, angst-filled teenage me could see that. "Maybe I could be a model," I said to my mother. "Sure," she said, clearly disapproving. "Perhaps next summer, when school is over, you can show them to someone." A year after the accident, we stumbled on those photos in a drawer. Now that I had a caterpillar of scarred skin crawling down my arm, it seemed ridiculous to imagine that any agency would be interested in such damaged goods. My mother, I felt, was secretly relieved.

It angered me that people saw me as ruined. I hated the scar. It carried the weight of tragedy. Yet even then I also knew my scar was a symbol of my survival. The surgery that put it there had saved my arm. After a year of physical therapy, I was once again able to stir pasta, dance, throw a football, and, in countless other ways, be a normal American teenager.

Later, in college, I would learn how to cover the scar with pancake makeup and powder. The director of a campus play I was in worried that my scar would be distracting, so someone in the theater department offered to help. Night after night, she covered the scar with stage makeup. Onstage, I was liberated. I felt like another person: not just a character but another me, one who didn't have a scar. By the end of the run, I had learned to put the makeup on myself.

After I revealed my secret to Josette, there was an interminable silence. I'm sure she registered my terror-stricken face. She glanced at my scar and then asked in English, "Have you seen a doctor about getting that removed?" Before I could answer, she waved away her own question with a dismissive *"Bien, bien."* This was a first: someone, and a modeling agent at that, who didn't care about my scar.

Santiago brought me to Spanish *Elle.* They admitted me, looked him over with a who-the-hell-are-you glare, and told him he could go. He waited for me outside. I was led into a room filled with many closets' worth of clothes hanging on garment racks. Editors snapped Polaroids of models, pinning the photos to a giant corkboard. The photos captured the models from the neck down only. There were no faces. We were fitting models, one step above clothes hangers. It was cold outside, but the clothes on the racks were sleeveless. The shoot was for a summer story.

To the girls, who were from all over the world, the editors communicated in polite but abrupt English. "Here," one said to me. "Put this on." I took off my sweater and peeled off my leggings and socks. I was conscious of my scar but even more embarrassed by my expired pedicure and my unshaven legs, stubbly and covered with ash, chalky against my brown skin. (Come on, who actually shaves their legs in the winter?) If I'd had my wits about me, I would've at least stopped at a drugstore for some moisturizer. I stood there, shivering and mortified, as these arbiters of beauty got a close-up of a regular girl.

Next to me another fitting model stood, awaiting her instructions. She was lithe and smooth with long, shiny blonde hair. She looked like she had just stepped out of a Breck Girls ad, her eyelashes curled, just a hint of makeup on her fair skin. She smiled when she saw me, a sunny, empty smile that revealed perfect white teeth.

Among themselves, the editors spoke Spanish, which at this point I couldn't speak a lick of. I had no clue what they thought of me. They smiled only after they'd dressed me, to admire their own handiwork. After a few hours of dressing, standing around, and undressing, the Breck Girl and I were dismissed. They told her to come back the next day. They thanked me for my time. At first, I shrugged off the rejection. This had all been too good to be true. I wasn't model material anyway. I had a pretty face, but I figured my skin color and scar put me altogether out of the running.

Still, part of me yearned to experience the glamour of modeling. But since it seemed impossible, I decided right then, full of delicious self-righteousness, to focus on higher things, like my education. *I don't want to risk lowering my GPA for some modeling job anyway,* I told myself. I wanted to graduate with honors. But the rejection stung. It would have been better if I had never entered the offices of *Elle,* never gotten a glimpse of the world I was now being shut out of. To my mother and grandparents, education was the most important goal for a young woman. But my response was self-protective, too. It's easy to scoff at a club that won't have you as a member.

Yet despite the certain-to-come embarrassments and rebuffs, something inside me had changed when Josette shrugged off my scar. Maybe it wasn't the deal-breaker I'd imagined it was. And though I hadn't been asked back to *Elle,* I did get a check two weeks later for twenty thousand *pesetas* (roughly two hundred dollars in 1992, if memory serves). In two hours, I had made enough to cover two weeks' worth of living expenses. Where I came from, you couldn't make that kind of money without a graduate degree and board exams. I thought about the degree I'd have in a few months—major in theater arts, minor in American literature. That piece of paper would have cost my family close to a hundred thousand dollars, more if you counted how much we would pay in interest after I settled my massive loans. All that money and I couldn't envision what I'd be qualified for, other than temp work. So when the agency, despite my embarrassing first outing, decided to take me on, I was thrilled. Between classes, I'd go on casting calls and get the occasional job, thanks to the surprisingly supportive Josette. I was competing for jobs that paid a thousand dollars a day. All I had to do was stand there and suck in my stomach. All of a sudden, I wanted very badly to be a model.

I sheepishly told my professors about my gig, and to my happy surprise, they encouraged my foray into Spanish professional life. They pointed out that being among Spaniards and having to interact in Spanish was great for my education. I enjoyed this new justification, so I left out the part about most of the other models being Swedish or German, most of the editors speaking impeccable English, and hardly any of them saying a word to me the whole time.

For a while, I girded myself for the inevitable disappointment I imagined lurking around the next corner with an "I'm smarter than this anyway" shtick. That evaporated with my first big gig during Cibeles Madrid Fashion Week. No high-minded snobbery about being too smart for modeling could negate the fact I couldn't even grasp simple directions. Sometimes I'll leave acquaintances with the impression that I became an international sensation right away, because the truth makes me wince.

At rehearsal, although I felt strange and shy parading around, scar or no scar, I was confident about the task at hand—the task being, well, walking. I was a sharp girl. I considered myself well read and articulate. Sure, these were the days before models just had to walk in a straight line. And sure, the instructions were given in rapid-fire Spanish. But following the simple choreography—synchronized entrances and exits, a few turns and crosses—should've been a cinch. And yet for some reason, when all the other girls walked right, I walked left. When they walked left, I walked right. After an hour or two of my screwing up, the choreographer said I could leave. *Phew, I'm done rehearsing,* I thought. I needed to recoup. I'd come back the next day and show them how it was done. Nope, I soon found out. I could leave, as in leave and not come back.

When the semester ended, I left Madrid, returned to Worcester to walk for graduation, then moved back home to L.A. with boxes and boxes of stuff but no game plan. After my glamorous European stint, I was back living inside the peach-colored confines of my old bedroom, sleeping on my mattress-and-box-spring-on-the-floor bed beside a bookcase filled with *Sophie's Choice, The Outsiders,* and *The Satanic Verses,* with its original red-bordered dust jacket.

I knew little about the modeling industry in the U.S., though I had seen a woman featured on the local news whenever there was a segment on models, which in L.A. was quite a lot. Her name was Nina Blanchard. I scribbled that down, then called 411 for the number. When I reached the receptionist for the Nina Blanchard Agency, she informed me they held regular open calls. I told my mom. "That's great, Paddy," she said, ever my booster. "If you want to go, you should go."

The forty miles from my mother's house in La Puente to Nina's Beverly Hills office felt more like four thousand as I drove from my lower-middle-class suburb into mansion land. Clutching my slim portfolio and wearing a hideous dress with big white daisies, I walked right into the office and waited. After a young and smiling Frenchman named Philippe saw my photos, I met with Nina herself. This time I'd come prepared for my audition. I wore short sleeves to avoid the awkwardness of having to bring up the scar myself. And of course I shaved my legs.

I didn't know it at the time, but Nina was the epitome of the iconic old-school Beverly Hills agent—the raspy voice, the Estée Lauder look, the commanding air. I always imagine her wearing a Chanel blazer with a big brooch. Nina, who passed away in 2010, was the Eileen Ford of the West Coast, the woman who made Cheryl Tiegs and Christie Brinkley, who launched the California blonde look. She was an institution.

She warned me that I wasn't in Europe anymore. My scar could be a serious obstacle. But she was willing to represent me. I couldn't have been more astounded if she had sprouted gossamer wings and pulled out a magic wand. My journey had begun. Elated, I planned to return to the agency after a two-week trip to New York.

Before my meeting with Nina, I had done a little homework and made ambitious plans to weasel my way into all the big modeling agencies in New York. I would be in the capital of advertising and fashion, roaming Madison and Seventh Avenues, so why not storm the offices of Eileen Ford, John Casablancas, and Wilhelmina? Nina advised me not to. I wasn't ready, she told me. I obeyed. In those days, you had a "mother" agency who groomed you and helped you build your modeling book of tear sheets from magazine editorials, and then that agency sent you to other markets they thought you could work in. They placed you at a sister agency and shared the commission.

When I returned from the East Coast, I set off on a Friday for a meeting at Nina's agency, this time with proud mom in tow, to meet the rest of the team and receive my marching orders. Nina wasn't there that day, but her head of fashion, Jack somebody, was.

He explained gingerly that my scar was not exactly a draw for editors and casting directors. "We have to think of our bottom line," he said, as my elation faded and dejection replaced it. Eleven minutes into my big meeting, I was headed back to the San Gabriel Valley. My mom was livid. "That scar is not your fault," she said, with tears in her eyes. But any anger I might have felt took a backseat to my sense that modeling in Spain had all been a fairy tale. I couldn't blame a modeling agency for being superficial. That was their business. All I understood was that in Spain, I was a woman, beautiful and confident. Back home, I was a young girl again, uneasy with herself, scarred, and brown.

I wallowed all weekend; then on Monday, as soon as I knew her office was open, I called Nina and explained what had happened. She said that she would keep her word, as I had kept mine while in the Big Apple. Nina fought with Jack. She was the owner, after all, and she ultimately took me on.

I wasn't expecting to be on the cover of *Vogue*, but I'm not sure I understood that the jobs I'd get would be commercials. My first job was a Folgers commercial, shot in L.A. but for the French market. I played one of several coffee groupies, wild for a caffeine-drinkin' man. For most of the day I sat around and chatted with the other models. They regaled me with stories. One had just done a video with Prince. Another went on about modeling in Europe—not "second-tier Europe," as she condescendingly referred to Madrid, but in Paris and Milan. How fabulous it all seemed! After three days of essentially lounging around, I left with a really cool pair of jeans from the shoot and $3,600—*cash*. I had never seen so much at once. I folded up the bills and crammed the wad into my front pocket. One girl looked at the bulge with an eyebrow raised. "Why don't you put it in your purse?" she asked. "Because I want it close to me," I said. I liked the feel of it against my thigh.

Nina was a motherly presence in my life. When jobs or castings ended late, she'd insist that I stay the night in the spare room at her lavish Mission Revival–style villa in the Hollywood hills. She didn't want me driving home late. I'd never seen a house like hers. I ogled the Spanish tile, the turrets, and the spiral staircase. Her stunning lawn had no curry leaf or kumquat trees, like my mom's, but I remember taking note of the St. Augustine grass. Peter had had a gardening business when he first arrived in the U.S. and St. Augustine grass, he always said, was the most resilient.

When I had both an early-morning and a late-afternoon call, Nina would let me hang around the office instead of having to trek home only to trek back later. On those days I'd bring lunch in a little Igloo cooler and eat in the conference room. In an office full of lingerie ads and tape measures, I must have made for a strange sight hunched over a Tupperware filled with one of my college staples: Top Ramen stir-fried with curried flank steak. I've always felt like a truck driver trapped in the wrong body. Today, I eat straight from pans with my fingers. I overturn blenders, the dregs of sauces sliding slowly into my mouth. Home alone, I get in bed, perch a pizza box on my lap, and go at it, wiping my mouth on my sleeve.

On the day a flamboyant Italian casting agent named Luigi came to the office, I had just polished off one of my favorite lunches at the time: approximately half a loaf of bread layered with tomatoes, basil, and mozzarella and doused with olive oil and balsamic vinegar. I'd just sucked down my last bite, fingers still greasy, when Luigi and Nina walked into the conference room. They sat down with a stack of portfolios. Luigi, I overheard as they flipped through them, was a scout for an agency in Milan. I quietly packed my stuff and had gotten up to slink out when he looked at me and asked, "What about her?"

I was no longer the girl who'd shown up ashy for a casting. I had confidence. I knew how to hold my body, and how to walk. My dark features would work in Italy, he thought. They certainly didn't serve me well in the U.S. Commercial work was about selling products. And the logic was, you'd only buy the shampoo if you identified with the model lathering her hair in the shower. His agency would front the money to ship me to Milan and put me up in an apartment his agency kept for models. I'd pay them back from the work I did. Nina, to my surprise, said no. She said she wanted to save me for Paris. I had no idea if she really had this in mind for me or if it was some negotiating technique. Either way, I decided to go. I yearned to be somewhere where I felt beautiful and sophisticated, as I had in Madrid. And at the very least, the opportunity meant I could finally move out of my mom's house in La Puente, the same old Carver-esque working-class neighborhood I had lived in throughout high school and that I had tried so hard to escape. The things I had seen and sampled, not only from my time in Madrid but also from rubbing shoulders with the many international students at Clark University, had left me thirsty for a more cosmopolitan environment. And although Worcester, Massachusetts, had been no London, Paris, or even New York, I had still been at an academic institution devoted to learning, close enough to NYC that I could drive or get there by train on the weekends.

Once I was discovered by Luigi in Nina Blanchard's office, I didn't look back. One thing I knew: I was not going to move back in with my mom, ever. I would do whatever I needed to, to make my own way to a life for myself. While in Spain, I saw for the first time a world much larger than my mother's or Peter's immigrant existence. My mother loved the theater and museums, but after moving to La Puente we rarely went to any. I can remember only once going to a musical that had traveled from Broadway to Los Angeles, called, ironically, *Sophisticated Ladies,* composed by Duke Ellington. From the time I arrived at JFK at age four until we left for California in the early eighties, my mom and I had gone to many Broadway shows, including *I Remember Mama, The Wiz, Chicago, Evita,* and *Ain't Misbehavin'.* My mom would wait in line in the cold for discount tickets, somehow managing to find the pennies from her nurse's salary to pay for all those lovely excursions.

I wanted museums, plays, and, most of all, a place where there were lots of people from different backgrounds who would inspire me and from whom I could learn. I hoped I could make a living in Milan, but, more important, I hoped somehow that even if the modeling didn't work out (which I had serious doubts it would, what with my scar and all) I would find a path that was right for me. I had gone to L.A. with little more than a BA in theater arts and a modeling portfolio, and after just a summer of pounding the pavement, it was pretty clear that opportunities for a girl like me were more elusive than they had been in Spain. I was eager to get back to Europe, where the notions of beauty and sex appeal were not as narrow.

I arrived in Milan on October 6, 1992, just as its status as the center of the fashion world had nearly completed its descent. I'd be staying in the south of the city, far from the attractive center and well into the gray, sleepy industrial section. Luigi's agency put me up in a building called La Darsena—Italian for "the dock"—appropriate, since it was the first port of call for new models in the city. It was like a low-rent version of the Barbizon Hotel, a repository for the thin and wayward. I had two roommates: a chirpy Brit who seemed more interested in men than in castings and a seasoned American model with a been-there-done-that attitude. At the time, it didn't occur to me that if she were actually as experienced as she acted, she probably wouldn't have been sharing a one-bedroom apartment with two other girls. They slept on two twin beds. As the new girl, I was stuck with the sleeper sofa in the living room. Good thing I stayed in Milan for only three weeks. Yet its unglamorous beginning didn't extinguish the thrill of my new life. No longer was I a moonlighting student. I was living with other models, because I myself was a real model.

Three days after I got there, Luigi and Chicco, his club promoter friend, told us to get ready, because we were all going out for dinner. I remember asking whether we would be going somewhere expensive. If so, I'd politely bow out. My English roommate laughed. "I've never seen a bill," she said. Several cars pulled up in front of La Darsena, and a gaggle of girls filed out of the building, teetering on heels, and piled in. My roommates were there, along with a twenty-year-old from Australia, a nineteen-year-old from Germany, and a sixteen-year-old from Omaha, who I remember thinking should've been at home with her mom. At hardly twenty-two, I was the oldest of the bunch.

Dinner was at a pizzeria. This I was excited about. I had never met a pizza-related food I didn't like. English muffin pizzas, stromboli, cheese-filled calzones, those gloriously greasy New York slices I had for lunch, seventy-five cents and worth every penny. We sat down and instead of Sprite, my typical pizza partner, we drank Chianti, deep red and tannic, with more weight than the Ernest & Julio Gallo that my mom bought by the jug. Before we ordered, waiters arrived with bread, crusty and warm; little bowls of almost syrupy olive oil that tasted of grass; and shards of Parmesan, like uncut diamonds. Before that night, I had thought Parmesan was a salty powder that came in a green shaker with a yellow top.

These shards were altogether different, studded with crunchy crystals and sweet with a funky dairy tang that overtook the back of my mouth like *chaatpati.*

I attempted to order pizza with pepperoni, siren of many a lapsed vegetarian. Yet when my pizza arrived—a whole pizza, nearly as big as my dinner plate, just for me!—I found it covered with marinated peppers. This was my first lesson in Italian. Here, *peperoni* meant bell peppers. The lack of spicy meat wasn't the only difference between the irregular circle in front of me and the massive triangles I'd scarfed down in the States. While I expected pizza sauce, pasty and dark, I was met with a glorious, warm, pulpy liquid the color of a summer tomato, which lightly coated the pie. Rather than a golden ocean of cheese on top of that, there were just milky-white tidal pools dotting its surface. And just as I was about to pick the whole thing up, I looked around to see my tablemates going at their pies with forks and knives. One bite and I knew: this was the Chanel of pizza. I had only ever known the Gap.

Around midnight, after demolishing the pizza and draining too many wine bottles, we crammed into the cars again and pulled up in front of Chicco's club, Madame Claude, named for the doyenne of the eponymous Paris brothel. Chicco led us as we strode in, a parade of thin, tall girls from all corners of the earth. We passed the waiting hordes, proud of our access and unaware that we were being sacrificed to the modelizers inside.

We were led to velvet couches and, as if out of nowhere, our intoxicants arrived. We danced with one another, careful to avoid eye contact as the vultures began to circle. But as the night wore on and the drinks kept coming—I'd had plenty of Chianti; I definitely did not need whiskey and Cokes—I turned into a vulture myself.

I spotted Luigi at a table chatting with two men and went over to say hi. I'm still not sure what came over me, but I turned to one of Luigi's friends, pulled his folded-up tie from his pocket, and wrapped it around my neck like a scarf. My impishness was innocent. At twenty-two years old, I had no designs on this man, unremarkable but for his resemblance to Michael Douglas (circa *Fatal Attraction*), mixed in with a bit of Al Pacino— but in *Dog Day Afternoon*, not *The Godfather: Part II*—and with about the same build. We danced all night and I reveled in the excitement of being in a new country, with a new, unknown life about to unfold. This was the first man in Milan who courted me, just three days after I arrived from the U.S., and he did it with charm and what I decided was the utmost panache. We met on a Thursday night and he asked if he could give me a tour of the city and show me around that Saturday. He showed up at the agreed time and when I got in the car he had everything planned for the whole day. I had assumed we would just drive around and have lunch and that would be it. We walked in the center of town and he took me to see the Duomo. Then we went to the artists' district of Brera to the Pinacoteca, to see works by Caravaggio, Raphael, and Rubens, but also to his favorite gelato place on Via Solferino. He took me to see designer boutiques I had only read about in *Vogue*, and then to a fast casual sandwich shop called Panino Giusto. He savored highbrow treats and lowbrow treats with equal gusto and filled our day with a mix of both.

My Italian beau, Daniele, and I would spend much of the next six years together. In Daniele, I saw so much of what I sought to be myself: he was worldly, sophisticated, and knowledgeable about art and culture. From the first, he had a huge effect both on my quality of life in Europe and on how I saw myself. I had arrived in October with one large suitcase of clothes and two thousand dollars, and that was it. By December, with the weather growing cold and my funds dwindling, he could see that I needed a bit of sprucing up. Daniele very sweetly bought me a cashmere coat with a fur collar trim, one that I sorely needed. I had left my puffy jacket and my wool coat back in the States. In fact, in those first days after college I still didn't even know the difference between a jacket and a coat. Daniele had lived in New York and spoke English well, so he corrected me. A coat, he said, went at least to the knees, whereas a jacket was only sport-coat length, hitting at the thigh, or even higher, around the hips, like a baseball or leather bomber jacket. That was where Daniele's tutoring started, but there was way more he would school me in over the years. I spent most of my twenties in Italy, much of that time with Daniele. I had never experienced a life like Daniele's. His family had very deep roots in the textile-making community of Como, in northern Italy. He had had a very privileged upbringing and while he was a bit of an overgrown, spoiled rich kid, he did also work very hard. He partied the same way.

In the world of fashion, much of the 1990s was a period of excess and debauchery for many of its inhabitants. And when you spend your time being judged for your body and nothing else, you sometimes need to leave it. Or abuse it. I began to dip my toe into a world I could not have afforded or even fathomed just a short time earlier. My healthy fear of hurting my mother or my relatives in India kept me from ever developing a serious drug habit, but I was not immune to testing the limits. I felt uninhibited, free to experiment and do things I normally wouldn't do. I wanted to please Daniele as well. But only I am responsible for my actions, not anyone else, and there are certain nights I'd rather forget.

I was eager to be an adult. I was not very experienced sexually, and when I wasn't sober, I felt free to do things I wouldn't normally do. It was the first time I had acted out my curiosities and fantasies. Some I regret, but not all, like knowing what it's like to touch and be touched by a woman. Not since I kissed two boys in one afternoon during a seventh-grade field trip to an amusement park had I been that promiscuous.

But these bacchanalian evenings happened only once a month or so. Daniele's appeal lay more in how much he made me laugh. He had a fantastic sense of humor and a playful childlike streak. He was very creative and a good singer who played the harmonica like a pro and loved to dance. He dressed sharply but in the understated Milanese uniform of jeans, blazer, crisp monogrammed shirt, and a simple Rolex. To be honest, a lot of this was lost on me at first. I didn't even understand how much Rolexes cost. In fact, I wouldn't have even been able to tell a Rolex from a Casio until he once pronounced that every well-dressed young woman should have a good watch, like a Rolex. He very sweetly gave me one on our first Valentine's Day together. All I remember thinking was that this small piece of stainless steel and glass had cost more than my mother made after taxes in a whole month as a nurse. I was terrified I was going to break it. And at first I wore it only when I was around him.

Admittedly, it did not take long for me to get more and more comfortable with this new flashy life, in which I traveled back and forth from Milan to Paris for the weekend (I moved to Paris two winters in a row to build my book) and down to Sardinia in the summer, where Daniele's folks had a house in Porto Cervo. But it wasn't just how to dress or the lifestyle or that Daniele taught me which fork to use (which he did!). It was also the many excursions he took me on to Florence, to Venice, to Rome. Daniele definitely was a hedonist, but he also had a serious, bookish side. He was a voracious reader and understood so much about European art and history. It was a joy to hop around Europe and experience all these things firsthand. I was totally wide-eyed and savored every minute of all the schooling I was getting. I worked only a few days a week, and often took a trip or two a month, getting an education that four years at Clark never gave me.

I was coming from a pretty humble existence, and while college did expose me to the way others lived, I had been a financial aid student who was right back in her mom's house after graduation. For me, modeling was really a chance at sophistication, at becoming cultured and getting to see the world in a way I would never get to otherwise. Daniele's choosing to be with me also seemed a badge of sorts. He had lots of choices and he had even invested in a modeling agency (not mine, though—I had the good sense to keep my autonomy there). But he wanted to be with *me*. Being rejected early on at all those modeling castings was tough. Daniele was the perfect salve. In a way, Daniele gave me the courage to feel like I even belonged at those castings, scar and all. In less than six months, I had gone from living with my parents after college and wondering how I was going to pay off all my student loans to going to La Scala, shopping at Kenzo, and eating at Bice. My head was spinning.

My years in Europe shaped me as a woman. I don't really think any of us are women right when we turn eighteen, or even twenty-one for that matter. You have to live a little. I certainly tried to do that. It was amazing just to walk the streets in those cities. There is so much history in the buildings alone. In Paris, I studied how French women dressed, so casual yet put together and nonchalantly sexy, so individual and idiosyncratic somehow, even if they all shopped at the same stores. I studied the way Italian women walked, so feminine and playful, to some indecipherable beat that gave them both poise and sex appeal at once. I was fascinated by the culture all around me.

And I explored those two cities through my fork as well. In Milan, the brioche and other pastry in the mornings, always with cappuccino, suddenly made me a sweet-eater. The pastas and meat dishes you could get at trattorias for a modest sum were simple in their preparation but deliciously complex in the mouth. I learned the regional differences between north and south and savored all the glorious seafood of Liguria. I never ate any fish until I got to Italy. Fish was the last frontier for my newfound carnivorousness to conquer. The first couple of years in Milan and Paris were surreal. I was in my early twenties, far from home in a new and exciting atmosphere with the freedom to really look at who I was and who I wanted to be. I had grown up in a pretty conservative environment in my mother's home. My stepdad wouldn't even let a boy talk to me on our front lawn in broad daylight. I was not a rebellious teenager in high school and was too worried about how much college was costing us to even risk jeopardizing my place thereafter. In Europe I was alone, without my parents or family, so I made my own decisions, and for the first time in my whole life money was not a constant issue. I wasn't making that much in that first year or two as a model, but compared with what my parents and I had to live on, I barely needed to work a couple of days to meet my month's expenses. It was an unbelievable turn of events in the history of my short life.

chapter 7

I joined a new agency that sent me to Paris to build my book after just one month of being in Milan. The apartment I lived in, on Rue du Chemin Vert in the Bastille neighborhood, was no better than the one I'd left behind in Milan. I shared two rooms with four other girls, all models, all wretched, in debt to our agency for rent and the pittance they advanced us for living expenses, and on a seemingly impossible hustle for work to pay it off. I went on endless castings and "go-sees" (where you'd go to see an editor or photographer in the hope that they'd take a shine to you), clutching my modeling book as I waited in line with two hundred other girls, only to have the kingmaker in question flip through my book without so much as looking me in the eye. I'd race from one go-see and casting to the next. At my low level, sometimes you'd get a job because you were the first hireable girl to arrive.

But at least I was in Paris. At least after I left castings dejected I could walk through the Place Vendôme or Jardin des Tuileries, admiring the city even if I didn't feel a part of it. The endless castings forced me to experience Paris by Metro and by foot, to wend my way through immigrant neighborhoods, past slivers of restaurants selling goat curry, down alleys packed with Chinese shops selling tea, ginger, and fresh cilantro, even in February. I'd scurry by butcher shops, averting my eyes and wishing I could unsee the skinned rabbits and lambs hanging in the windows, eyes still in their sockets, or the pigs' heads, each wearing a strange smirk. I had only just started eating meat a few years prior, and, as far as I was concerned then, it should only come nestled in Styrofoam trays and wrapped in plastic.

To buoy my spirits, I spent the little money I had trying to buy a small piece of Paris through its food. While I couldn't really afford to eat out very much, I could afford to roam Paris's markets and cafés if I watched my budget. Just a hunk of cheese with good bread and olives were all I needed. Cheese and olives smashed between the flanks of a crisp baguette was the perfect combination of umami and *chaatpati* in one starchy, crumbly bite. The spicy-sour spike in the various olives I found, from small black oily Greek ones to big chili-drenched Moroccan ones, was the perfect salty counterpoint to the fatty and sharp cheeses of France. I wasted nothing. If the heel of the baguette became a bit dry, I would drizzle drops of the seasoned brine or oil from the olive bags on top to soften the bread.

There were endless varieties of cheese to sample. Week by week I slowly made my way from the mild and familiar to the more sinister, stinkier, runnier sections of the cheese counter. It was in Paris that I first discovered goat cheese, or chèvre, by accident. I had eaten the chived-up cow's-milk cheese Boursin, which is sold in American supermarkets, and thought that's what I was buying when I pointed to the creamy mound in the cheese shop. But instead of the cream-cheesy, soft richness of that herby wonder, I discovered the sublime, grassy tang of goat cheese! Before that my only taste of goat cheese had been Greek feta. I was in love with French cheese.

And so I made friends with the large, sweaty cheesemonger in the Bastille street market, who would bray at me with raised fingers on his shiny head for goat's cheese or pull imaginary teats for a buttery Brie de Meaux. This tall, paunchy man, a doppelgänger for Alfred Hitchcock in a tablecloth-sized white apron spread across his enormous belly, had huge, wide hands with pink sausages for fingers. The broken capillaries on his cheeks and nose bulged as he barked at me to stop loitering and fogging up his glass case. Often a swarming knot of irate French housewives and maids formed behind me while I tried hard to pick just one cheese. There were so many to choose from, and so few francs with which to buy them. Back home, at the Amar Ranch Market, we basically had the choice of mozzarella, American singles, or Wisconsin mild, sharp, and extra-sharp cheddar. For spaghetti we sprinkled Parmesan out of a dark-green Kraft cylinder. If we went to the Stater Bros. supermarket farther out in West Covina, which was slightly more middle-middle-class than the lower-middle-class La Puente, we could score Swiss, provolone, and Muenster. French cheese to us was Laughing Cow. Cheese was either white or orange. But in Paris, in the Bastille, cheese was blue, beige, veiny, creamy white, yellow, deep sunset orange, or even burnt sienna. It came crusted with rose-colored peppercorns, smelling of funk, and swathed in ash and wax.

My love of cheese was liberated. I perused and savored all the milky delights I had never before seen or tasted. As weeks went by, my French improved ever so slightly, and I would stammer questions at the impatient beast of a cheesemonger. To preserve his business from dwindling, he took to pushing me to the side in order to service those who *did* know what they wanted. Because I was probably pathetic and because he could most likely see the hunger in my eyes, often while cutting a wedge for those sharp-elbowed women, he would throw a razor-thin slice or crumbled edge my way. He never looked at his hands while wielding his knife or sharp violin string of a cheese cutter. And yet the amount was always perfect. He was not kind and he was not chatty, but if I stood there quietly, he would ply me with a steady stream of cheesy samples. "So what wins the prize today?" he would grumble, to indicate he had given me enough.

Some days, if I was especially lucky, he would give me the leftover scraps of cheeses that were too small to sell, even in the bargain basket of four- or five-franc wrapped chunks. I took whatever he threw my way, and eventually relished even the most intense Roquefort or the runniest Camembert, waxy rind and all. I didn't have more than eight or ten francs to spend on any given meal. One day, the agency's unhappy accountant called me in to discuss my purchases. After what might have been the first talking-to a model has ever received for eating too much cheese, I slunk out, chastened and worried for my Camembert habit.

Thank goodness, then, for Michael Spingler, from whom I learned the principles of French cooking. He was a French literature professor at Clark, and while I'd never taken a class with him, his wife, Kathy, worked as the costume director for the theater department and had employed me as a costume apprentice. I adored her. Michael happened to be in Paris on sabbatical, working on a book about Molière. He knew I was struggling and had me over for dinner often. Michael showed me a Paris different from the one I'd seen, which was beautiful but cold and full of disappointment. His building was in the 14th Arrondissement, at 139 Rue D'Alésia, if memory serves. The building's owner, Jean Claude, was a literary critic for *Le Monde;* its handyman, a German poet. They were all friends with Leo, the owner of a nearby bookstore called Alias. Everyone except Leo lived in the building, for the most part with their doors open. Jean Claude, a tall man with approximately ten hairs left on his head, all white ones; wire-framed spectacles; and a small roster of moth-eaten sweaters, would show up for dinner with a pot of beans and lardons. Michael would make magic with his two-burner stove. It was there I ate my first *blanquette de veau* (my first veal of any sort, for that matter), the French bistro classic that featured the slowly cooked meat doused in a sauce rich with stock and cream. I ate lamb shank braised in red wine, and nearly everything—steaks, green beans, fish—was finished with plenty of butter. In Michael's hands, even the simplest food became special. We did not eat mere mashed potatoes. No, we ate *purée de pommes de terre.* He'd make Jean Claude peel the potatoes. "Jean Claude was in the army," Michael would say. "He won't mind."

To come back from those dispiriting casting calls to the heady aromas of his tiny kitchen, or to Michael and Jean Claude sipping wine beside an ashtray brimming with the butts of unfiltered Gauloises cigarettes, was exactly what I needed. To climb the wide marble staircase to the fifth floor and enter the spacious apartment crowded with tattered furniture, dusty oriental rugs, and miles and miles of dog-eared books to see these two thinkers semi-drunkenly discussing Baudelaire was a much-needed balm for my aching feet and spirit. I'd kick off my high heels, sink into a chair, and receive a glass of red and a warm welcome. "And how was today's foray into the forest of fashion?" Jean Claude might say in heavily accented English, exaggerating his Fs.

Michael and Jean Claude saw the toll that the fashion business was taking on me and they fought it valiantly, deploying a daily barrage of gentle teasing. When I came in crushed after failing to score a commercial modeling gig, probably a half page in some newspaper insert, they expressed mock disappointment in me. "How terrible you are!" Jean Claude would say. Michael would chime in: "I agree, you're definitely not good enough to sell Maalox." They'd poke fun at my self-pity. "One day, your grand moment will come," said Jean Claude. "You *will* have your face on the pantyhose package at Monoprix." I had my own peanut gallery. That is how I survived the parade of rejections inevitable for most wannabe models and the myopia of a young person's passion. They reminded me that there was more to life than being pretty.

I spent more and more time on Rue D'Alésia as my apartment became bedlam. One day, I came home to find that someone had drunkenly peed in my bed. I was paying for a soiled bed in an apartment I rarely used. I cried when I told Michael. He invited me to move in. This was when my real life in Paris began. Work came in a trickle—a fitting-model gig here, a catalog shoot there—but the occasional job was all I needed to support my modest lifestyle. I certainly wasn't partying like a model. When my former roommates were out at Les Bains Douches, the French equivalent of Madame Claude, guzzling free champagne with other trucked-in models, I was with my weeknight family—Michael, his friends, and, when they came to visit, Kathy and their two kids—eating coq au vin and drinking pinot noir. When the weekend came, I was off to Milan to see Daniele, or "Monsieur Spaghetti," as Jean Claude dubbed him. I was living as charmed a life as anyone sleeping on a literature professor's couch could hope to. Michael and Jean Claude used to heckle me as I packed my bag. "Going away for your dirty weekend?" *No!* "Well, isn't he your lover?" *Ew, stop!* As embarrassed as I was, I felt grateful to have these two paternal men in my life who felt protective enough to embarrass me.

I got to know the Friday-night pilots, who would let me sit in the cockpit's third seat for takeoff and landing on the short flight to Milan. They'd point out the rabbit holes near the runway at Charles de Gaulle, and curse the rabbits for getting caught in the wheels. The airport staff was occasionally invited to hunt them. My pilot friends boasted of the stews they'd make. When I landed back in Paris on Sundays, I'd look out the window for the animals' eyes, glowing from the reflected lights of the plane.

Daniele's mom, Gabriella, a big-bosomed, always carefully coiffed woman with a weakness for furs and skinny cigarettes the size of lollipop sticks, opened my eyes to a sort of Italian cooking much different from the spaghetti-and-meatballs version produced by Pompeii Pizzeria, the restaurant run by my friend Pelly Dimopoulos's family, where I had my first job at fifteen. (In those days, you could get an age waiver at fourteen from the Department of Labor to have a part-time job after school.

If your grades were good enough, the school would sign a document and you were exempt from waiting until the legal age of sixteen to work.)

I watched, surprised at first, as Gabriella opted for butter instead of olive oil and often chose béchamel over tomato sauce. I had received my Italian food education at Pompeii Pizzeria and, a year later, at Pelly's uncle's pizzeria, Mario's, where the tips were better. There garlicky tomato sauce reigned. Yet Daniele's mother mainly cooked the style of food found in northern Italy and Milan in particular, which meant risotto tinted yellow from saffron and rich with marrow, accompanied by osso buco slowly cooked with white wine and stock. Somehow it reminded me more of French food than Italian. When we went out to eat, they would discuss whether to go for food from Emilia-Romagna, Tuscany, or Liguria, as my friends and I back home might debate whether to eat Chinese, burgers, or Mexican. I knew Indian food was highly regional, but India was a vast country of close to a billion people. I quickly learned that Italy, though comparatively tiny, had no less regional variation. Daniele's family was full of voracious eaters. Before I'd taken a third bite of my veal Milanese, incredibly juicy and encased in crispy breading, they were sitting in front of empty plates, watching politely and with evident pride as I savored every buttery moment.

Between Gabriella and Michael, I got a vast education in European cooking. I learned how to make more than just curry and stir-fry, to cook without relying on mountains of chopped onions, garlic, and ginger. Occasionally I'd pitch in to do more than chop onions. In February I came home giddy from the supermarket, because I'd found fresh cilantro. Michael was roasting a lamb shank for dinner, so I made an almost-but-not-quite replica of the cilantro chutney of my childhood, to drizzle onto the meat.

Daniele spoke perfect English, but taught me to speak real Italian, in the way only a boyfriend can. When we met, I spoke enough Spanish to piece together what Italians said to me. Within a few months, though, I could fight with him in rapid Italian. Through our life together and from chatting with cab drivers, I came to understand both the expressive and the banal. *"Che cazzo!"* a cabbie would yell after getting cut off. *"Ce lo mal di stomacho,"* Daniele would say right before chugging Maalox.

About once a month, Daniele and I would spend an entire Sunday at the movies—we'd have lunch, catch an afternoon movie, have a snack, then see another film, and after that we would eat dinner before a late show. These weren't all Roberto Benigni films, of course. For years, I thought Steven Seagal was an amazing actor, because the guy who dubbed him in Italian was a brilliant stage actor who also dubbed De Niro. Daniele lived near the Duomo, the city's stunning cathedral, and we often walked past it on our way to the movies. There was no ornate cathedral adorned with thousands of centuries-old statues back in La Puente. There were no skyscraping Gothic spires, either. Daniele cultured me in the way a partner often does: in the person you care for, you often see parts of the person you wish you were. In Daniele, I saw a man raised around what I knew cerebrally to be great art, the kind you read about in college. He knew it not as something to be studied but as something to be seen and felt, and not as something rare to be viewed only after a long plane ride but as something beautiful that happened to be right down the street. That proximity to art and culture was part of what I had missed when we moved away from New York. Now I had a chance to live walking distance from Santa Maria Delle Grazie, where *The Last Supper* hangs. I was a train away from both Michelangelo's *David* in Florence and the Colosseum and Pantheon in Rome.

From Daniele, I learned so much about Italian food, in the quotidian way you do when your days and nights together are full of pumpkin ravioli swimming in sage butter. He meticulously planned our movie times and snacking. Pre-movie lunch might be at Pizzeria Gambarotta, then after movie number one, *spuntini* at the luxe café Cova, its ceiling dripping with chandeliers, for little sandwiches of arugula, goat cheese, and leathery bresaola (cured beef) or some pastel-colored pastries fit for Marie Antoinette. I loved eating in tiny portions, the opposite of my experience in America. Even my Coca-Cola came in a miniature glass bottle. After movie number two, we were off to dinner at Il Rigolo, the Tuscan trattoria we went to every Sunday and possibly the only place in the world to offer *lasagna al curry*. This cracked me up, and I ordered it often, a béchamel-heavy stack of pasta stained yellow with turmeric. Only occasionally did I look for these reminders of home in my food. For the most part, I embraced the new and unfamiliar, in the way you do when you're young and captivated by a life different from the one you've known. I did, however, order my *pasta arrabbiata* as angry as they could make it—for an Indian girl, their "spicy" was never quite enough. Somehow our favorite lunch in Milan during movie days was at the nearby McDonald's—ah, Italy, where modernity and antiquity exist side by side—where I'd lay into *un Big Mac* and a side of *patatine fritte.* Somehow even McDonald's was better in Italy.

Besides treating his money-strapped girlfriend to fine food, Daniele also upped my sartorial game. Textiles were his family's business and he had his own operation, making and selling printed fabric. He did "research" constantly, by which I mean he shopped. I'd tag along for his sessions, where he'd buy whatever inspired him and send it to the fabric factory for a few days to be studied and some aspect of it replicated. He'd always buy whatever it was in my size, so after he was done with it, I'd get to wear it. He had great taste. I had my own style, a hodgepodge of vintage bargains and a few splurges from Contempo Casuals and Express, but he gently challenged my choices. He taught me the subtle and not-so-subtle precepts of fashion, the unspoken rules that no one had ever codified for me. A very short skirt and heels were overkill. If I liked a sweater or pants, he'd politely check the tag to identify the fabric. This isn't good quality, he'd explain, or this won't keep you warm. Daniele made sure I had the staples. Just as a good home cook needs to have high-quality olive oil, nice vinegar, and a heavy sauté pan, a girl needs a dress coat, real leather boots, and a nice watch. And just as it's impossible to go back to cheap balsamic after tasting the good stuff, it's hard to slip on rayon once you've worn cashmere.

Three months into our relationship, he took me for the weekend to the Swiss ski resort St. Moritz, where his family had a house. Our first night there, he hired a horse and sleigh to drive us across the frozen lake. With snow-capped Alpine peaks in the background, he proposed to me. As romantic a gesture as this seemed to be, and as doe-eyed as I was, I had no problem saying no. I was naïve, not stupid. I cared for him, but I was too young to marry anyone, especially someone—and goodness knows I see the comedy in this now—seventeen years older than me. In fact, marriage didn't figure into my girlish fantasies. From my mom's three marriages, I inherited a skepticism toward the institution, with its "till death do us part" commitment. I promised to marry him one day, adding "if all goes well" so I had plenty of wiggle room. That's how I said no. And so the relationship sailed on, ultimately for six years, as if nothing had happened. I was in love and just happy in the way you are when you're young. The future felt far, far away. Commitment is easy before a relationship requires compromise and obligation. I felt wise then, proud of my man and his sophistication, the complete opposite of my mother's latest choice in a mate. Somewhere inside, I knew it wouldn't last. The relationship was one, ultimately, of contented convenience. We stayed together because we were reasonably happy and because there was no good reason to split up.

A year had passed since I arrived in Europe and not much had changed. I was making ends meet, with the huge help of having no rent to pay when in Milan, but the work had become increasingly tiresome. I was no stranger to rejection by this point. There were several explanations for this: I wasn't a particularly gifted model. The waif phenomenon was in full swing, and I was a (relatively) voluptuous 34-24-34. Yet I couldn't help but see all those nos (or, more accurately, the lack of any response at all) as a referendum on my scar. I was bored of the shame I felt, of people's furtive downward glances when I went sleeveless, of the inevitable questions the scar invited. I was tired of the requisite disclosures when I went on castings: "Before we begin, let me show you my hideous scar." I saw an obvious ceiling to my achievement.

I accepted that I would get only so far with my aesthetic handicap. So I made an appointment to undergo chemical dermabrasion to take some of the dark pigment out of the scar. This wasn't the first time I'd tried to reduce its visual impact. Before I had cold-called Nina Blanchard's agency, I'd visited an Indian surgeon named Dr. Raj Kanodia in L.A. recommended to me by another model. He told me that while he couldn't erase the scar, he could significantly flatten it, making it easier to hide with makeup. This might be uncomfortable, he said, before inserting a needle as long as an asparagus spear and withdrawing it excruciatingly slowly to ensure an even distribution of Kenalog. The injection did flatten the scar but left me terrorized. Now, after a year in Milan, my agency identified a doctor—agencies had Rolodexes filled with doctors who could fix anything from teeth to tits—who treated it inch by inch as I gritted my teeth and cried. This was primitive dermabrasion—essentially a controlled chemical burn, a painful stripping of layers of tissue—which I hope has improved since the early nineties. I had never known such agony, even during painful monthly periods and in the car accident itself. But the procedure worked. After a dozen sessions, about half an inch of the scar had been visibly pruned of a few layers of knobby tissue and was now a neutral color, close to that of the rest of my arm.

My agency sent me for a go-see with the agent Davide Manfredi, who was looking to cast the next photo series for a photographer named Helmut Newton. Art lovers, fashion-industry types, and *Vogue*-magazine devotees—they all knew Helmut Newton. I'd first heard of him when I was in college. In the same league as Irving Penn and Richard Avedon, he was a trailblazing photographer who made his own rules. Mr. Newton urged fashion photography from the restrained toward the provocative— a big deal at the time for a demure industry. (A *Vogue* editor reportedly admonished him: "Ladies, Helmut, do not lean against lampposts.") He was perhaps best known at the time for the series *Big Nudes,* unflinching, elegant portraits of women who were completely nude but for a pair of high heels. Being chosen as his subject was a potentially career-making job.

When my turn with Davide came, I entered his office with familiar trepidation. He told me to strip to my underwear. I was neither surprised nor entirely comfortable. I had been modeling for a year and was more or less immune to the humiliation of being photographed in this state. It had become only mildly unpleasant, like getting blood drawn. At least by now I knew enough to shave first. As I undressed behind a partition, I gave him my requisite scar spiel, half expecting him to tell me to put my clothes back on. "Don't worry, Helmut likes scars," he said. He took a few Polaroids, affixed them to a piece of paper, and faxed them, along with hundreds of others, to Mr. Newton in Monte Carlo.

The audition came and went. I thought little about it, because I did not for a second expect to get it. I was a benchwarmer for my agency. Once in a while, when a job came in that wasn't commercial, they called me in to take a swing. I had a better shot at scoring that kind of job, where the model would be a subject of art, rather than a consumer aspiration. While an ad exec would not see my "exotic" look as relatable, the artist might at least see it as fun to photograph.

My career so far had been an elaborate game of pretend. I was a model who barely got work, who existed on the lowest rung of the business, and who saw no indication of that changing. I was still effectively in debt to Luigi for the plane ticket to Milan and to City Models in Paris. Somewhere in me I understood that the farce would soon end and I would move back home, go to grad school, find a real job. As a result, I was only partly present during my auditions and shoots. As I stripped for Davide, I felt as if I were role-playing, as if I were looking through someone else's eyes.

Two weeks later, I got a call from my agency. They informed me that Mr. Newton wanted to book me for a private commission. Me! Perhaps the coolest part: he loved my scar. The minute he saw it, Davide later told me, the great photographer said, "I have to photograph her." My agent was thrilled, of course, almost shocked. Everyone at the agency seemed genuinely happy. The underdog had won one. I was an MFA student getting a story in *The New Yorker.*

This could be the job that launched me from an unknown model with a funny name to a model with a funny name that bookers recognized. Instead of being just one of three hundred models on a casting call, I'd be one of forty. If I was able to say I worked with Mr. Newton, it would no longer matter that I wasn't the most beautiful or talented model in the business. Once you graduate from Harvard, does anyone really care about your GPA? Get through this, my agent promised, and I could forever sport his imprimatur. The subtext for me was that my scar, that indelible blot on my body, would be effectively erased.

Once the excitement faded, I began to confront what the shoot would entail. Mr. Newton, I learned, had been privately commissioned by a Japanese businessman to do a sort of *Big Nudes* redux. It was not to be published or exhibited but merely hung, perhaps in his dining room. I'd have to be naked. To get a sense of how naked, Daniele and I went to a bookstore to look at Mr. Newton's work. As I flipped the pages, I understood that this was not "strategically placed fabric" naked. It was full-blown, oh-my-that's-your-vagina naked. I was terrified of posing completely nude. I was a child of conservative India, where women went to the beach in their saris. My grandfather was still alive. He would not be happy. I also hated the idea of a photo of my poontang hanging in some banker's dining room. This was an odd reaction, I now realize. But for some reason I'd rather have had thousands of people staring at my body than just that one.

Vag was the final frontier, the thing you still didn't see on TV or in mainstream ads and media. Italian magazines like *Max* and others did show fully nude models, and many respected Italian actresses and TV personalities had gone full frontal by then, some more artistically than others. Later, I would do *Max* magazine, but that was still to come. At that moment in time, in 1993, just showing my boobs with both nipples blazing seemed like a crossing of some Rubicon in itself.

My body tensed as Daniele and I leafed the pages of one of the Newton books. Daniele noticed. "You should only do it if you're comfortable," he said. "If you're not, it'll show." He was right. You can fake being bubbly for a Folgers shoot. You can fake the obligatory stoic look of the runway. But when you're entirely exposed, the camera won't be fooled. And I couldn't go all the way to Monte Carlo on this legendary photographer's dime to be a disappointment.

Yet whenever I thought I'd finally decided to demur, the infectious thrill among my colleagues and my agency pulled me back into "maybe" land. Perhaps I was just nervous. I didn't want my fear to torpedo such a huge opportunity. I spoke to my mother, who has never been prudish. She had raised me not to be ashamed of my body, and to appreciate the female form and celebrate it. We both routinely went naked around the house when there weren't others around, and I never saw my mom behave as if she were ashamed of her own body, no matter what. We even went to a nude beach once in San Diego, when I was an adolescent, mostly out of gleeful curiosity but also because my mom and I did like being naked. I mean that we just liked the naturalness of it. At Black's Beach we quickly became bored after seeing that most of the other beachgoers were older gay men. Any shred of feeling risqué or sexy because we were nude on that beach quickly evaporated. My mother understood that posing nude could be a celebration of the female form, not just the culmination of male fantasy. Yet as the days crept forward, my doubt grew. Two days before the shoot, I got into my bed and called my agent. Exasperation barely concealed his fury. No one says no to Helmut Newton, he said. I had embarrassed the agency and myself.

A few weeks later, I got a surprising call from my modeling agent. Mr. Newton was shooting a calendar for Lavazza, the Italian coffee company, and wondering, what if I wasn't completely nude, but just topless? Not only hadn't I blown my moment, but I didn't have to compromise in order to grab it. I was glad and relieved they still wanted to work with me, especially as I was still feeling a bit like a chicken for turning the other job down, especially at the last minute. The atmosphere in Milan at that time in the early 1990s was much more liberal than in America. Italy (Catholicism notwithstanding) was much less puritanical than the United States, and overt images of female sensuality and sexuality were much more prevalent in magazines and on TV. Women with fully nude breasts nursing infants in commercials for baby bottles or formula were commonplace on Italian TV. It was also a time before the Internet. Things you did in photos couldn't haunt you and follow you in the same way.

More than exploitive, the atmosphere seemed to be one that celebrated the female form and equated breasts with femininity and motherhood. Often all but the cracks of buttocks were exposed in thong bikinis, and on beaches along the Mediterranean and Adriatic Seas, grandmothers and teenagers and everyone in between bathed and sunbathed topless. Even excursions in Sardinia with Daniele's family proved eye-opening. So the compromise, the willingness to show my breasts, seemed an easy one. I mean, if even Daniele's mom could go topless then surely I could, to work with an artist like Helmut. I didn't regret refusing the first job with him, but I was left with a feeling that I had missed a great opportunity, not only for my career, but also as an artistic experience. At that time, as now, pretty girls were a dime a dozen, and most of them didn't have the extra handicap of being brown or having a scar seven inches long down their arm. Retouching was still not an option for almost all but *Vogue* covers back then. Models poured out from every residence and hotel. Milan was the first stop while building your portfolio, and if you didn't want to do some job, there were lines down the block of starving girls who would, with a smile.

The other motivating factor was that this time the job was not for a private commission, but for a Lavazza calendar! Lavazza is one of the oldest companies in Italy. Like Pirelli, they commissioned great photographers to shoot an annual pictorial calendar. So I guess the coffee company didn't require full bush! Not only would I not have to put my nether regions on display, but people would also actually see my work with Newton.

Daniele drove me to Monte Carlo. The shoot was in a suite at the Grand Hotel. When we arrived, I went upstairs, and Daniele sat on the hotel patio reading *Corriere della Sera*. I reached the suite only to find that one of my closest friends, Antonio Gazzola, had been booked as the makeup artist. His presence was a good omen. In those early days, he was somehow always there at the right moment. Backstage, he used to whisper to me in Italian that I was just as beautiful as all the other models and that my scar made me special. He knew how anxious I was about the scar and would tell stylists they didn't have to worry about putting me in short sleeves, because he would make the scar disappear. Of course, they always put me in long sleeves anyway.

Now, though, he left the scar alone, because Mr. Newton didn't mind it—or so I'd heard. Antonio was finishing up when Mr. Newton came in to say hello. He treated me gently and kindly, as a grandfather might. He spoke about his wife, a comfort to a girl about to spend an hour topless with a strange man in a hotel room. I began to feel at ease in my own skin. Then he caught a glimpse of my arm. "What have you done!" he gasped.

I began to panic. After the agony of turning down his first offer, the thrill of a second chance, and the years of wondering whether my scar was a deal-breaker—whether the accident had permanence—Mr. Newton's reaction could be the ultimate rebuff, the moment at which my wondering whether I could make it as a model was met with a definitive "No, you cannot."

"Didn't they tell you about my scar?" The words barely escaped my mouth. "Yes, yes," he said, "but why have you erased a part of it? You've ruined the beauty of it. Antonio, get your paints out and restore that mark to what it was." I couldn't believe it. I can still remember Antonio smiling with a brush between his teeth as he touched up the scar, adding wine-colored lipstick to the lightened areas. "Crazy business," he murmured under his breath. While I was there, Mr. Newton booked me right away for another project. In these photos, my scar, not my boobs, was front and center. I felt so comfortable with this man, so safe. And when I posed for a picture for *Big Nudes 2*, you could see only the side of my face in the Polaroid he showed me. The scar was the star. The Lavazza calendar I wouldn't see for ages yet, but he did send me a print of my own of the *Big Nudes* portrait.

Antonio knew what I didn't: when the designers found out I had shot with Helmut Newton because of my scar, not in spite of it, they would all want to use me. Already grunge was in, and models with tattoos and piercings were showing up in American ads for Calvin Klein, and Europe often followed America's lead. Helmut would give everyone in Milan and Paris the courage to use me without camouflaging my scar, Antonio said.

He was right. And it helped, I'm sure, that my agent milked the shoot for every drop—oh, did I mention that she just shot with Helmut? That he loved her? That he rebooked her on the spot? I was soon booked for an eighteen-page shoot for Italian *Elle* and I shot Roberto Cavalli's first campaign with Aldo Fallai. I was booked for many shows in Paris, from Ungaro to Sonia Rykiel. At the shows stylists still checked my sleeves— but now they were checking to make sure the sleeves were short, so that everyone would know who I was under all that makeup.

Bigger jobs presented more opportunities to improve as a model. I learned how to walk from the legendary modeling agent Piero Piazzi. "You walk great," he told me, before essentially advising me to change everything I was doing. I shouldn't move my shoulders or my head. Just my hips. I had been overdoing it, walking the way my young daughter does today when she pretends to model. Gradually I got better at the strange craft of modeling. I learned to hold my body in a nonchalant way for editorials in that nineties grungy attitude that seemed to be screaming, "I *don't care* if you take my picture." I learned to move in a way that made the clothes swing and look fun on the runway. I also began to understand how to make my body seem slimmer and longer in lingerie and swimsuits on film. My growing success came in part from Mr. Newton's photos, but also from my newfound confidence, which his embrace provided. All of a sudden, agents at castings were excited to see me. The spring in my step showed in my work.

For the next four years, I lived most of the clichés that come with modeling success. There I was partying on yachts, going to conspicuously cool restaurants, and heading to Ibiza for the weekend. I'd awake on a boat with Daniele, parked near just a few others in the Mediterranean Sea, and go to the prow wearing only my bikini bottom. I knew that men and women on the other boats might see me. And if I knew someone was watching, I might turn so my scar was visible. My scar became adornment, like a string of pearls. Almost overnight, it had transformed from a stain into a sort of talisman, a source of power and confidence.

Today, I love my scar. It is so much a part of me. I wouldn't remove it even if a doctor could wave a magic wand and erase it from my arm. I've started seeing my body as a map of my life. I can tell a story about every imprint life has made on my skin: the mosquito bites on my back from when I slept under the Sardinian sun the summer I first fell in love with Daniele; the scrapes on my leg from the rocks in the Cuban sea during the filming of my first movie. In her introduction to *Women*, by Annie Leibovitz, Susan Sontag asks, "A photograph is not an opinion. Or is it?" I believe it most certainly is. A photograph can change the way you look at yourself, though it's more complicated than that. Perhaps it was under the right light, or through the right lens, that I really saw myself for the first time. I have Helmut Newton to thank for that. People have told me that my scar makes me seem more approachable, more vulnerable. Ironically, the greatest gift fashion has given me is the courage to expose that most vulnerable part of myself. By facing the shame of my own body's disfigurement, I was able to liberate myself from that shame, and instead draw confidence from my scar.

chapter 8

I never decided to stop modeling. By 1997 or so, I was getting bored and less and less ambitious. I would work only if I needed the money, but I had no healthy desire to really make as much money as I could. And it's hard to get anywhere with modeling if your look goes out of favor with fashion and its trends. I was not a waif. I once got fired from a Sonia Rykiel show because I gained too much weight between seasons. I was bored and it seemed modeling was bored with me, too.

Fortunately, another career began to take shape. Because I was a foreigner who spoke Italian—a relative novelty—I was a sound bite favorite of the news crews that covered the fashion shows for the style-conscious Italian media. Eventually, RAI television asked me to join the cast of *Domenica In,* Italy's version of the *Today* show. I asked the director about showing my scar on TV. "Everyone knows that you have a scar," he said. "Don't cover it up." I spent every Sunday for six months on live Italian TV in Rome and lived the rest of the week in Milan. The show provided a sort of training ground for every TV job I've done since. Each live show lasted six hours, and it aired without even a five-second delay. The anxiety this induced motivated me. I could finally make use of my mind. Sure, I was more Vanna White than Katie Couric, but at least I finally had a job where the goal wasn't to shut up and look pretty. Plus, these were those heady pre-Internet days when a slipup wouldn't make it around the world in a matter of hours. No one from back home would even watch the show.

The producers played up my role as the screwball-comedienne foreigner still learning the language. I had my own segment on the show called *Parole a Parole* (Word for Word): I had to attempt to provide the definition of a difficult Italian word and an elementary school student would get to guess whether I was right or wrong. In my dressing room, I had hundreds of letters from kids vying for the honor. The producers loved that sometimes my Italian would fail me. By then, I could speak the language rapidly and intelligibly. I just happened to speak a strange pidgin dialect that was part cab driver—my unofficial teachers—and part profane fashionista, thanks to Daniele and his friends. This occasionally made for exciting television. When one of the show's other hosts teased me on air, I teased back, attempting a gentle insult like "jerk" but accidentally using the word *stronso*, which essentially means "piece of shit." The slipup earned me a clip on *Blob*, the Italian version of *Talk Soup*, a show so popular it spawned a verb—*blobato*, as in *"Mi hanno blobato!"* ("They blobbed me!").

Soon after, a film agent signed me on and cast me in an Italian costume drama set in Cuba at the time of the conquistadors. They needed an "exotic girl" who spoke a bit of Spanish to play a Cuban native. Never mind that I had gone from the high-art world of Helmut Newton to a period piece that had cast a Tamil woman as a Cuban "savage" (topless in a loincloth, though I insisted that they give me hair extensions that would cover my breasts). Never mind that the peoples who populated pre-Columbian Cuba didn't speak Spanish. I couldn't exactly be picky—this was my first acting gig, five long years after graduating from Clark with a degree in theater. I was thrilled.

More roles followed, including another in a miniseries where I played a swashbuckling Malaysian princess from the nineteenth century, and a guest role on an Italian TV series with Nino Manfredi where I played a character that IMDB dubbed "Indian lady." I hadn't made it big, but I did feel like I was making it. I loved being on the set with the PAs and cameramen and grips, the hairdressers and costumers and producers and directors. I loved that our prepacked lunches included a small plastic container of red wine, like those little plastic juice cups with foil tops they give you on airplanes. (Even craft services are better in Italy than anywhere else.)

I liked acting better than modeling for a number of reasons. It was more stimulating, but beyond that, it didn't feel like a blatant exercise in selling something. I wasn't exactly doing Shakespeare in the Park, but for the first time since college, I felt the satisfaction of coming together with others, all of us with the same script in hand, bringing to life something bigger than any one of us could achieve on our own. The best modeling and photography does tell a story, of course. But with acting I felt that I had the chance to tell a story that unfolded, to be a part of a narrative that changed over time and provoked in the viewer a myriad of emotions, beyond the brief reaction provoked by a still image. I also loved meeting so many talented technicians on the set. I was curious to learn about how they approached their work, and I wanted to learn from them how I could be better at mine. My director on *Domenica In*, Michaele Guardi, taught me as much about improvisation as I had learned in four years of college.

So when the Food Network offered me the opportunity to host a show, I jumped at it. I had just published my first book and was eager to figure out what to do next. Even though it wasn't an acting job per se, it was about food. I couldn't wait to get back on a set. Little did I know that slowly, while waiting for that big break in acting, I'd actually become good at the work I'd found I loved. The experience I had on *Padma's Passport* and then *Planet Food* would later be topped by *Top Chef*, which would wind up being the perfect mix of the things I loved: travel (we went to a new city every season, and another for the finale), food (I learned from the best), and hosting on television (something, that, by the time I started, I had ample practice at). Part of what I love so much about the *Top Chef* experience is that because it travels from city to city, much like the movies I filmed, the set really feels like a big circus: an improbable place built quickly out of nothing, and just as easily dismantled and stored for the next adventure. It's especially unlikely given how complex the set is.

The *Top Chef* set is divided into two major parts. There's the part you see on camera—the kitchens and Judges' Table, and other sights like the pantry sporting the *Top Chef* logo—and there's the part you don't see. Wherever we're filming, whether we're in the desert or the rain forest, the production staff sets up a control room, or, as we all call it, Video Village. Video Village is where the elves work. Magical Elves, in fact—or at least that's the name of the production company that puts on the *Top Chef* circus. These are the people who make the show the success it is.

Video Village migrates depending on the shoot location each day. It winds up in some pretty janky places: an alleyway near a Dumpster, a muddy field, a parking lot next to a construction site. If you show up on the set and wonder why there's a tent in the middle of the sidewalk, you've found Video Village. Inside, there's a low hum. People sit and hunch in front of laptops and tablets, jotting down time codes and snatches of dialogue for postproduction. Audible above the hum are the voices from the shoot, emanating from the monitors: Tom critiquing a sauce; the contestants fretting in the Stew Room, where they sit and wait before we send one of them home.

There's a bank of a dozen or so monitors, each showing a different setting or angle. Two people always sit in front of the monitors, staring at them and talking, it seems, to no one in particular. The most vocal of the two is Paul Starkman, *Top Chef*'s director and resident mensch. At the bottom of each screen in front of Paul is the name of a different camera operator. Like a high-tech puppeteer, Paul controls filming by calling out their names followed by his instructions, his eyes seemingly everywhere at once.

"Send them in, Brenda," says Paul, and he watches one of the monitors as the chefs trudge single-file toward Judges' Table. "Give me Emeril. Okay, zoom in. Stay on Brook, she gives a better reaction. Look at that, Tom's taking tickets! That's so good, Eric! Give me Padma. *Padma.* PADMA! God damn it!"

In this way, the story line takes shape. As Paul gauges the unscripted judge and contestant reactions, he looks for theater in truth. Paul hears John Besh say, "That's a very difficult dish to pull off." In that line, Paul sees a dramatic element, snapping his fingers and exclaiming, "That's good!" When a contestant stands out, in a way that's good, bad, or both, Paul lets it guide him. "Is Dale the story tonight?" he might wonder aloud.

Next to Paul is the show's executive producer, for the past several years a woman named Nan Strait (although we've had several others), who is the little voice in my ear. While Paul commands, Nan quietly guides me. I hear her often in my earpiece, helping me play effective host and occasionally protecting me (and therefore the show) from myself. I might be sitting beside Tom or Wolfgang Puck when my must-prove-I-belong-here reflex kicks in and I take a stab at culinary erudition. Suddenly, there's Nan to tell me, as only she could, "Padma, save it for PBS," or "That was great, but three million people just changed the channel."

She's also there to remind me that not everyone at home knows all the food words we're tossing around inside our little bubble, where we all know the difference between brunoise and julienne. When I launch into praise of the African spice called grains of paradise without identifying what the heck it is, I hear Nan bringing me back to the real world.

"All right, for those of us cowpokes who watch the Super Bowl and make Velveeta nachos," she says, as gently as she can, "can you explain what the hell grains of paradise are?" When I do, Tom, not knowing I've been instructed to hold forth, looks at me like he wants to fillet me. I'm not telling *him*. I'm just looking at him while I tell the people at home.

Sometimes keeping my lips moving is part of the job. In my efforts to steer or maintain the conversation among judges to please the producers, I often embarrass myself. I awkwardly toss around cheffy terms like "expediting" and "pickup time." I pronounce someone's rendition of the root vegetable salsify delicious while pronouncing the word "salsif-eye" instead of "salsif-ee." (I've also at various times rendered quinoa as "kin-oh-ah" and calcium as "cal-shum," thanks to the many accents and languages in my head competing for access to my mouth. Realizing I'm mispronouncing a word always makes me cringe. It's even worse when I do it in front of Thomas Keller and fourteen rolling cameras.)

Nan goes through the scripted parts of the show with me, not just to give me extra practice, but because some of the wording must be very carefully followed. *Top Chef* is technically a game show and therefore governed by FCC regulations. The contestants are supervised at all times. Their phone calls are monitored. If a contestant talks to me off camera, a producer jumps in to say, quietly and seriously, "Please step away from the judge." The tone is such that you almost expect him to follow with " . . . and put your hands behind your head." The slightest whiff of collusion is a no-no. I'll be on the set, gabbing with a producer, and I'll hear "Chefs within earshot!" Any talk about the show stops immediately. I'll be in the bathroom stall and I'll hear, "Chef walking!" as a contestant comes into the bathroom with their escort. Who knows, the thinking goes, whether or not I'm on the pot talking to Gail on the phone about a recipe?

Occasionally, the only filming going on is of the chefs in the kitchen. That's when I like to visit Video Village to watch the cooking happen in real time on the monitors. Even though the chefs are typically working in a giant professional kitchen, the scenes conjure for me the solitude and quietude of cooking at home. The soundtrack is more familiar, too: the low buzz of silence broken up by the occasional slurp, clinking of spoons, rustling of cotton, the tinny scraping of whisk against bowl. It's a testament to the skill of the producers, cameramen, editors, and the rest of the production team that the show is such a thrill to watch. Because without splicing, cliff-hanging commercial breaks, and music, the footage can be decidedly unexciting. Unexciting, but lovely, too, the happy tedium of cooking on display.

Whether you have an office job or one on a television set, the days and years pass and the next thing you know, the people you were thrown together with by chance become more than colleagues. Time fosters connection. And over time the people on *Top Chef* have become a sort of second family to me. After I moved out of the home I had shared with Salman, I felt totally rudderless, but the show gave me something to hold on to. It was a real thing that I could be proud of and count on when I had little else. I felt immense gratitude to have a job that required my full attention, so that I was forced to set my personal heartbreak aside, even if only for the duration of filming.

It was the same summer of my divorce that the show received its first Emmy nominations. It hadn't really occurred to me that that might happen; it wasn't even on my radar. But in some important way, our show being taken seriously by the Television Academy made me take myself more seriously, made me sit up and take notice of my own work. Until that point in my career, I had mostly waited for the phone to ring, for someone to give me an assignment, whether it was modeling, writing, acting, or hosting. Awards aren't the reason you do things, or important in themselves, but the Emmy nominations were a turning point—I went from hoping things would work out to seeing that they *were* working out. *I am actually doing this*, I thought. *Maybe I'm not just flying by the seat of my pants.* I didn't want to be passive anymore, personally *or* professionally. In that moment, I came into being as my real and present professional self.

Top Chef and its success gave me the courage to think proactively about shaping my career, and I began to explore what I wanted it to look like. For the first time, I began to consider my goals and my interests in a clearer and more pragmatic light. Until then, I had chased every lead because those were the only opportunities I could see. I had to publish two cookbooks and host three different food shows before I finally took my culinary hobby seriously and gained a modicum of true professional confidence. It had taken me well into my middle thirties to begin to come into my own, but no matter. I now had a direction to point myself in. I began to think about other work I would find rewarding that I could pursue when *Top Chef* wasn't filming. The greatest gift that *Top Chef* gave me was the blessing of living intentionally, with agency, and doing what I really loved.

chapter 9

I met the man who would change my life on an accidental date. Rick Schwartz (a movie-producer friend) and I had hatched a plan to turn Jhumpa Lahiri's Pulitzer Prize–winning collection of short stories, *Interpreter of Maladies*, into a movie. Rick set up a meeting with Teddy Forstmann, the chairman and CEO of IMG, the global sports and media company, who had deep enough pockets to fund several movies. I suppose to a different sort of person, his name would have at least rung a bell. Not to me. I didn't know anything about the world of private equity, mergers, and buyouts. If I'd owned a bird then, I'd have used the *New York Times* Business section to line its cage.

I didn't want to go to the meeting. I didn't feel I belonged there. After all, Rick was the brains behind the operation. He was the producer, the guy who understood deals and investment and distribution. But Rick insisted. Mr. Forstmann might wonder why a Jewish guy from New York wanted to do a film about Indian immigrants. I'd be there to preempt the question.

This was in early May 2007. Although my and Salman's attempt at reconciling had failed for good and we had decided—for the second time—to divorce, we were still living under the same roof and trying our best to be civil to each other. So I was actually in a cab with Salman when I called Mr. Forstmann's office to set up the meeting. Salman gave me a look when he heard me ask for "Mr. Forstmann." "*Teddy* Forstmann?" he mouthed, all arched eyebrows.

Salman's reaction made me feel like I should've known about this guy, Teddy. Later, Google filled me in. He had pioneered the leveraged buyout, borrowing money to buy companies, then refurbishing and selling them. He and his partners at Forstmann Little made a fortune doing it, and he owned a production company and had recently acquired the legendary talent agency IMG. He had dated Princess Diana. All of which sounded good to me, because we were trying to finance a movie.

The next day, I got a call from Teddy. We spent a while chitchatting. I remember thinking, *He can't be such a big deal if he's able to spend twenty minutes talking to me.* He was available to meet Sunday for dinner, which I thought was an odd day and time for a business meeting. "I'll pick you up," he said. I told him I could probably get there myself, thank you very much. "Were she alive, my mother would be upset if I didn't pick you up," he told me.

Whatever, I thought. *He's eccentric.* I'd just meet him and Rick at whatever restaurant Teddy chose. But two days before the meeting, I got a call from Rick. He had to be in Chicago for a movie he was producing with Tim Robbins. He couldn't make it back in time.

"No problem," I told him. "I'm sure we can reschedule."

"No way," said Rick. "Teddy Forstmann isn't an easy man to pin down."

"Then does it have to be *dinner*?"

"If he wants dinner, have dinner."

From Rick's urgency, you would've thought this Forstmann guy was the pope. I called his office to tell him Rick would be unable to attend the meeting. Unlike the few big businessmen I'd had brushes with before, whose secretaries handled all logistical negotiations, when I called Teddy's office, I got Teddy. I launched into my best impression of an important movie producer.

"Mr. Forstmann," I said. "My partner is stuck on another production. On Sunday, it will just be me."

"Great," he said. "Where should I pick you up?"

Dinner was mostly a blur. We went to Il Cantinori, a quiet, candlelit Italian restaurant in the East Village. Nervous and tasked with convincing this guy to back us, I managed to inhale my scaloppine while talking a mile a minute about the movie. With every sentence that spilled out, it became clearer to me that the man to whom I was hawking this niche film was the type who'd sooner fund a Spielberg blockbuster. There was nothing about Teddy that read "indie" or "niche." He used the word "neat" a lot. He seemed to me to be the epitome of the Establishment, the very white, very male majority who run corporations, the government, and the world. He wore a sapphire and gold pinkie ring with a crest engraved on the stone on the same hand as a Jaeger-LeCoultre watch.

Halfway through the main course, the conversation took a strange turn. "That house you live in, I only saw one doorbell," he asked. "Do you live there all by yourself?"

"No," I said, "I live there with my husband and stepson." I still had my wedding ring on, not yet ready to accept failure publicly. What's more, I had no designs on Teddy—dating any man was the last thing on my mind—and I did not want him to know that my personal life was anything but normal and happy.

"I thought you were separated," he said.

He had read a snatch of gossip about my marriage in a tabloid, a small dose of schadenfreude for the casual reader but thoroughly gutting to me. Apparently someone at the Waverly Inn had overheard a conversation about my relationship with Salman being over. As Teddy spoke, my stomach dropped. Not only was I being reminded about my unraveling marriage, but the very private fact was also being delivered by someone I barely knew. Then, after a moment, I understood: I was on a date.

"I thought this was a business meeting," I said.

"I thought it was odd that you were wearing your wedding ring on a date."

"Date? I'm pitching you a movie!"

"My dear, it's not that you aren't bright and *quite* a talker," he said. "But this is slightly below my pay-grade."

I felt like a fool. I hadn't understood the difference between an executive at IMG and the guy who *bought* IMG. Of course Teddy wouldn't have met with me about my little project. "I'll tell you what," he said, sensing my embarrassment. "You should meet with Rob Dalton, the creative director of IMG, before he goes back to L.A." The only chance I'd have to do so, he said, would be a few days later, when Teddy and Rob would be at Teddy's "box" at Sotheby's auction house. "I'll be selling some paintings," he mentioned offhandedly, as if he were telling me to drop by his stoop sale.

A few days later, I went to Sotheby's to meet with Rob. Because I felt duped about the nature of my first meal with Teddy, before I headed to Sotheby's I called Rick and read him the riot act over the phone. He insisted he had not sent me to the dinner for anything other than business reasons. I felt further reassured knowing there would be several people from Teddy's office at Sotheby's with him. I'd been to the great auction house once before with an art-dealer friend. We'd sat on folding chairs shoulder to shoulder with other dealers and spectators, watching paddles rise and fall. It was exhilarating, the slides of the great works up for sale flashing on the screen behind the podium, the auctioneer calling out the vast sums of money. I never did think to look up, above the action on the floor. But on the day I went with my assistant to meet Teddy and Rob I discovered that above the auction pit there are boxes where heavy hitters look on in privacy—people who make the strivers downstairs seem like commoners. When I arrived, Teddy was observing an auction for one of his Modigliani paintings.

"Come on, Junior," he joked many months later, "you were turned on by all that."

"Not at all," I said, doing my best impression of a wealthy dowager. "A man is much more attractive when he's acquiring than when he's unloading."

The truth is that Teddy mesmerized me. I felt drawn, not romantically but almost anthropologically, to his presence. His success, mysterious to me in its particulars until later, provided an intriguing subtext to every sentence and every gesture, however banal. Sitting in that box with Teddy, Rob, and a gaggle of their colleagues, I felt like I was watching Muhammad Ali have brunch. At Il Cantinori, Teddy had given me his full attention. Here, he was still a gentleman and unfailingly polite, but he handed me off to Rob with a mere sentence, something like "Rob, this young lady's got some big ideas. And a book about Indians in America." Rob took it from there. I tried to explain why a book of short stories on immigrant Indians in the U.S. would make a great movie. But it was hard to be articulate in that atmosphere. Teddy, meanwhile, was busy offloading a couple of Modigliani paintings! I couldn't understand why anyone would want to do that. Who was this strange creature in black tasseled loafers?

I mentioned to Teddy that I was soon headed to L.A. to surprise my mom for Mother's Day. How funny, he said. He would be heading to L.A. at the same time. "Would you like a ride?" he said, the way I might have proposed driving a friend upstate. I stared at him blankly, trying to figure out what the heck he meant. "On my plane," he added, sensing my cluelessness. I'd already bought my ticket, but I couldn't turn down a trip (my first ever) on a private jet.

Days later, I found myself at a heliport on the eastern reaches of Manhattan. The helicopter took us to Morristown Airport. When we landed, we exited the helicopter directly onto the small runway, then from there we boarded Teddy's Gulfstream V, a gift from the private-jet maker for buying, then reviving, the failing company in the mid-nineties. Just walked right up a small staircase and into the plane. No lines, no security, no taking off my shoes. It was exciting. I felt like a child getting on a roller coaster. Inside, instead of the rows of seats I somehow still expected to see, I saw what looked like a cozy living room outfitted with four big chairs facing each other, a small long bar with two crystal bottles of brandy and magazines, and a dining table with plush banquettes that seated four across from the bar. There were three flat-screen TVs total. Toward the back of the plane was another seating area—not the fully reclining seats some airlines sell to first-classers, but two couches that could each seat three and could collapse to become a proper bed, queen-size and plush. As Teddy got settled, I tried to play it cool. He had an apartment that could fly. I couldn't help thinking about my mom's first apartment on East Eighty-Third Street. The plane's cabin seemed about the same size.

Over thirty years had passed since I'd lived in that apartment, since I had first arrived in New York from India, which now felt more like several lifetimes distant. That flight from Delhi to John F. Kennedy Airport, which had been my first, had brought its own kind of wonder. I had been just four years old when my grandparents had put me on a plane, alone, to cross several oceans and continents. A journey that would reunite me with my mother, whom I had seen just once in two years.

When my grandfather left me at the Delhi airport that October morning, I had on shoes, not a typical feature of my wardrobe at the time, and a bright-red wool coat with a hood and a big bow just below the collar. I had never needed a heavy coat before. My grandfather, however, had been to America and knew true winter. Fastened to the inside of my coat was a glassine envelope containing a slip of paper with the address of my grandparents' house in Delhi—a sort of return address for me, a little red and brown package. Their phone number and my mother's information were also listed. I can still hear my grandfather reciting the phone number aloud, saying "naught" for "zero," prompting me to repeat after him. I was excited. I didn't understand where I was going or how long my trip would take. But I knew I'd see my mother again.

I flew Air India. The trip—the local-bus equivalent of air travel—took me from Delhi to Cairo, Cairo to Rome, Rome to London, and finally London to New York. I loved every minute of it. The plane's interior was baby blue and the stewardesses—the supermodels of the seventies—were impossibly glamorous, wearing large *bindis,* bouffant hairdos, and printed silk saris. They strode the jetliner's aisles, calling out, "Coffee, tea, juice!" in their poshly accented English. Between flights, I watched their saris flutter as they walked briskly down the jetways, each woman carrying a pink Samsonite beauty case.

I sat near the front of the planes, with the other kids flying solo. The stewardesses plied us with coloring books and little paper puppets of the airline's mascot, a mustachioed maharajah wearing a red Nehru jacket. One older girl who made the trip with me through many planes and airport gates wore plaits in her hair, bottle-cap glasses, and a yellow plaid dress with a ruffle at the bottom and a bow at her back—very Holly Hobbie. Her trip was traumatic. At the gate in Heathrow, I watched her throw up on the back of her chair, staring as the vomit cascaded down the polyurethane. I wasn't nauseous. I spent my trip marching up and down the plane aisles. I was excited to be flying in the sky, gazing at downy clouds outside my airplane window. I felt elated to be on my way to America, and to be reunited with that most glamorous and elusive member of my family, my mother.

I didn't know then, of course, that the crossing from New Delhi to New York was more than a crossing of oceans and continents; it was a crossing of cultures, of lifestyles, of ways of being and knowing. I would be debarking in a New World. I would never be fully at home in India again or ever fully at home in America. I couldn't have looked back, even if I had thought to.

As Teddy's plane rumbled into the sky and we settled into our chairs, the disparity between the lives we both had led really struck me. I had a sudden and strange realization: besides the pilot and two attendants, we were the only ones aboard. On that first trip with Teddy, the unspoken agreement of the commercial plane ride—talk minimally to your seatmates, if at all—did not apply. So our flight felt a bit like a road trip, just the two of us looking for ways to pass the six hours it took to reach LAX. We made a game of our conversation. We decided to go back and forth, sharing a story from each year of our lives. I began with my mother's first divorce and my decampment, my first flight, and our reunion on Halloween night. I told him of moving back to India a few years later, leaving out the most personal details, and then returning to New York. I told him about moving to L.A., modeling in Europe, and my forays in TV.

I found myself, for the first time in a long while, recounting my life to someone far removed from it. He was not part of my ever-overlapping worlds of fashion, food, or TV (as many of my friends were). He wasn't a writer, editor, or publisher (as many of Salman's friends were). He was unaffected by the Kool-Aid I had so eagerly drunk. I felt liberated of the self-seriousness that occasionally afflicted my industry's tales of TV shoots and casting calls. And unlike the Bombay-born Salman, Teddy had grown up in Connecticut. He listened to my Chennai stories with particular curiosity. I saw the strangeness of my peripatetic childhood and young adulthood reflected in his face.

He told me about his family, his childhood and coming-of-age, about how he'd supported himself with money he made playing bridge. He told me about his first job out of law school, as a prosecutor for homicide cases. We continued to trade stories until we reached year thirty-six, when I ran out of years. He had thirty more to go. I learned there was more to

Teddy than business deals. He told me about his friendship with Nelson Mandela, who had given him one of his prize possessions: a replica of the dish Mandela had eaten from inside his Robben Island prison cell, inscribed, "Best wishes to a precious and generous friend." He told me about his sons Siya and Everest, South Africans who had been orphaned, and whom Teddy adopted and adored. He told me about the children's charities he supported, leaving out information I'd later discover—that he had cofounded the Children's Scholarship Fund, to which he had given $50 million and which had subsequently raised more than eight times that amount. Besides that, he also worked with the Hole in the Wall Gang Camp and funded a couple of camps for kids with terminal illnesses. And he conducted an annual fund-raiser each summer for still other children's charities. Most people—myself included, at first—did not realize how copious his philanthropy had been. He preferred to give in a way that did not involve his name on the sides of buildings. "I've got monogrammed towels and golf shirts for that," he'd say.

Aside from the final hour of the flight, when Teddy began to excuse himself every ten minutes or so to make brief phone calls, we spent the entire trip talking. Later, he told me that what I thought were important calls to some CEO or board member were actually calls to his pilot, Tom Ritz. It turns out a Gulfstream V doesn't really take six hours to get to L.A. from New York.

"Ritzy," Teddy had asked Tom, "can you fly around the block a few times?"

"We're running low on fuel," Tom joked back. "Make your move already."

I did not fall in love on that plane ride. There is a myth about love, that it happens in an instant; that there must be a spark that generates immediate flames; that the flames must roar right away. When I met Teddy, I was in no emotional state to start a new relationship. I was still reeling from the free fall of my divorce. I had been as high on life as you could get—in love, happy with my career, confident as can be that it would all last forever—and then in no time, I was alone, nauseated and unsteady from the rapid descent. I approached Teddy with caution.

My divorce had highlighted the faults of my relationship blueprint. I was old enough by then to recognize that the principles that had guided my choice of men could have been pulled directly from the She Has Daddy Issues handbook. I never knew my father. Until my twenties I didn't even know what he looked like.

I did have a doting grandfather, however. My beloved K. C. Krishnamurti, or Tha-Tha. For more than three decades, he worked as a civil hydro-engineer in the Indian government. During his heyday, in the late 1960s, he managed enough water to control a third of India's power. He was so distinguished in his field that after a short tour surveying hydroelectric plants and dams in America and Canada, he was offered a much-higher post by the Canadian government. A devout Brahmin and vegetarian, he politely declined. He figured that as a manager, he'd be forced to entertain in his home and serve meat, which he was not prepared to do. Later in his life, when I pressed him, he admitted that he had also declined in order to spare his children yet another move. Despite his success, he was, like most government workers, squarely in the middle class at best.

He was born in Kerala in an enclave of Tam Brahms, slang for members of our Tamil ethnicity and our Brahmin caste. Our family home had long been up north, but when he retired at age sixty, in 1977, he moved the family back south to Chennai, the capital of the Indian state of Tamil Nadu, and then called Madras. He felt, rightly, that his pension would go further down south. He would also be closer to his relatives, to the ocean, and to the hub of *dosas*, the savory rice and lentil crepes made on iron griddles at the vegetarian tiffin halls near the Mylapore temple in Chennai. He often said, jokingly or not, that he wanted to die in the land of his forebears but still live in a city. So he arrived in Madras rather than Kerala, where he purchased the two-bedroom third-floor flat at A-7/5 in G.O.C.H. colony (Government Officers Colony Housing), in the neighborhood of Besant Nagar, where I would spend some of the most formative years of my life.

KCK had always wanted to practice law. His parents had nine children, so sending a son to law school was not in the financial cards for them. After a career as a hydro-engineer, he could handle the cost. So upon moving to Madras, at age sixty, he enrolled himself in Anna University to study law. After graduating first in his class, he worked as an apprentice to a younger advocate, and eventually took a case of his own, winning insurance money for a widow. He promptly retired from law and ran a tutorial out of our home in arts and letters as well as math and sciences. On Sundays, he tutored to any college students who couldn't afford to pay. Everyone knew KCK's flat in Besant Nagar. If you ever got lost going there, you needed only to walk to nearby Elliot's Beach and ask one of the many young men leaning on their scooters and having a cool drink. KCK's love of knowledge didn't relent even during the last few years of his life. When I'd come to visit, I'd find him at his desk, behind a stack of books. "What are you doing, Tha-Tha?" I'd ask. "Working out some physics problems, Pads," he'd reply. He wanted to keep his mind sharp.

Mornings of my Madras childhood smelled of steeping coffee, steaming tea, and sandalwood. I'd wake up to the sounds of my grandmother haggling with the vegetable vendor through the window and of water being splashed hard by the mugful on the cool marble tile of the bathroom. After bathing, my grandfather washed his own garments, wrung them dry, and hung them in the sun on a clothesline on the veranda. He would anoint his body—once a decathlete's but by then rotund, with a belly and a grand double chin—with stripes of sandalwood paste and *vibhuti* or holy ash, as would most Brahmin men. Then he'd comb back his receding salt-and-pepper hair with Brylcreem, Pat Riley–style. To this day, I cannot think of him without conjuring the combined smell of Brylcreem and sandalwood. While the women of the house chased after us to put on our uniforms and collect our books and tiffin boxes of hot curries and rice for school lunch, while we yanked on our shoes and socks and hightailed it downstairs before the bus stopped honking and left us in the heat and dust, he chanted his morning prayers and *slokas* on the veranda. Before the sun's heat had reached full force, he'd set off on his daily morning constitutional accompanied by his carved walking stick and the other retired attorneys in the neighborhood.

Of all the people in our family, no two had a tighter bond than KCK and me. He doted on me endlessly, and among his three grandchildren, I was his pet—at least until Rohit, his first grandson, was born. After my mother left for America, he took it upon himself to prep me for our eventual reunion. To my four-year-old self, it felt like I was an astronaut getting ready for a trip to the moon. Tha-Tha was my mission control and the senior officer who had made that voyage and come back to tell about it. He had traveled to the U.S. numerous times and gave me as much information as he could about the gravity and air on this new planet called America. He spoke of tall skyscrapers and of something called the subway. He said that children played baseball, not cricket.

When I met new people, rather than stay silent and invisible, he taught me to say, *Hello, how are you doing today?* In 1970s India, people preferred children to be seen and not heard. America seemed to require a gregariousness that was not lauded in our culture. Truth be told, he loved America and relished pouring all his accumulated knowledge into his first grandchild. Tha-Tha made me memorize all fifty U.S. states alphabetically.

He made me memorize the name of Gerald Ford, the U.S. president. He taught me to sing "Ol' Man River," a 1920s ballad from the musical *Show Boat*, about a dockworker's struggle against the great Mississippi River. He loved this song and sang it in a slow baritone, doing his best to approximate a black American's southern accent. The song was a metaphor for struggling against the currents of the river of life, as experienced by an African American stevedore in the Jim Crow south. I wonder if he feared that my mother and I would never be accepted as equals there. Would we be discriminated against like the African Americans he read about? To his very Indian way of thinking, education was the best defense against this, so he would educate me as much as he could on the ways and mores of my adopted culture and hope that it in turn adopted me.

He told me stories of how he navigated American restaurant menus to feed his vegetarian stomach in the land of meatloaf and chicken casseroles. He described cooking for his hosts during a business trip and teaching them to make yogurt rice, of their incredulousness at the possibility of not starving to death on just lentils and rice. They seemed to think that this was the cause of India's poverty, but he assured them that one could feed more people with the milk of a cow than with its flesh.

He spoke wistfully of buying hot coffee and a warm donut for fifty cents at lunch counters when there was nothing else he deemed suitable. He loved donuts. We had no Indian equivalent of a sweet that size. Soft and fluffy, filled with air and cottony starch, shellacked with a sweet white glaze or sprinkled with sugar and cinnamon dust, donuts were the thing he missed most. He talked of donuts reverently. Tha-Tha and his *sweet* tooth!

Tha-Tha focused a lot on the food in America. Food was, of course, central to his existence. You could tell by his big Santa Claus belly, which in those days I often slept on at night. But mealtime in the States was when he had struggled most. It was the one facet of American life he, as a Brahmin man, a lacto-vegetarian, could not totally assimilate to or fully enjoy. He told me to be very careful when I ordered food outside my mother's house because there was hidden meat lurking everywhere, even in harmless-seeming soups. You'd be ready to eat some gorgeous, shimmering-hot "vegetable soup" in the snowy Yankee winter, he'd warn me, and then just as you closed your mouth to swallow, you would sense a meaty odor in the broth, a dark, sinister flavor no God-fearing soul could consume. Even fruit pies or potato crisps, which I loved and ate by the handful, could be fried in the extracted and liquefied fat of an animal. They called it lard. I needed to keep to the side of the culinary road. I was warned to seek the safety of simple bread, butter, and cheese to sustain myself until I learned to decipher what was safe to eat. America was where anything could happen. A cowboy Wild West of freedom, vice, plenty, and charm, where the boundaries were different and much, much wider.

He knew what I did not. I would now be an outsider for the rest of my life. My parents' divorcing had made me one in India already. He wanted to arm me with as much information, to pad my insertion into the new world to come, because he knew that I had to become an American child. I could only hope to survive if I made that identity mine. And when I returned "home," to India, I would be an outsider there, too, because I had tasted the West.

I realize now that he must have lavished me with so much attention to compensate for the permanent loss of my father and the spells spent without my mother, and later perhaps because he knew the circumstances of my return. Regardless, his affections were in full force. And as they say, women often seek in their partners what they saw in their fathers. For me, my doting grandfather played that role. His were the qualities I came to crave, those of a mentor, an older, wiser man. Indeed, Tha-Tha was my first mentor. It seems to me now that over the years, rather than searching for other father figures, I perhaps searched more for other mentors.

Daniele was my second mentor, when I was a new model, fresh off the boat in Milan. Here was a man with money and choices, and he chose me. He was the perfect boyfriend for that period in my life, both cultural mentor and badge of my own worth. After my modeling career petered out, I started to crave approval for my mind, in many ways long dormant during my stint in fashion. Salman played the same role—times ten. My love for him was as real as it was for Daniele. But our emotional needs supply some of the kindling necessary for that initial spark. And whether you know it or not, they help define the at-first blurry vision of the man with whom you imagine yourself walking hand in hand. When I met Salman, I had just come off the ego boost of several years of modeling and cohosting a talk show with the highest ratings in Italy. Yet moving back to the U.S., I left these successes behind and essentially started over. I'd entered a much more competitive job market as a woman who was, by the harsh standards of show business, past her prime. My hard-won self-approval had begun to evaporate.

When I was a girl, my confidence came from doing well at school, a goal set by a family full of strivers with graduate degrees. While I knew KCK and my mother were proud of my success as a model, I also knew they expected more from the girl who idolized her high school English teacher and looked forward to Academic Olympiad meetings as much as most girls did school dances. As my mom always reminded me, whenever I sulked about some small failure in Milan or Paris, beauty is not an accomplishment. This was her way of comforting me by noting the arbitrary nature of the modeling world, where no matter how skilled you were at posing, walking, and talking, you landed jobs because of your God-given cheekbones and waistline. Yet I also knew that, while she was too kind to admit it, she had higher hopes for me.

Salman mentored my intellect. After spending my twenties grooming my outer self and my manners, I was ready to groom my mind. His love and support gave me confidence to pursue my writing in a way I might not have without him. I began writing for magazines, as well as signed a second book contract. I started to consider new endeavors, a jewelry line and a line of teas and spices. Before my husband, I don't think I would have thought I was capable enough to attempt those things—he had buoyed me up and been a considerable, if unwitting, cheerleader. The way Salman made me take myself more seriously was not dissimilar to how my body image changed when someone like Helmut Newton thought differently of my scar.

Surprise, surprise, Teddy was an older, more accomplished man. In other words, prime Padma bait—a worm to a fish, a fish to a bear, a mango to an Indian girl. This time, however, I wasn't biting, or so I thought. The recent failure that was my divorce had convinced me that I needed to change my patterns. So unlike Salman's, Teddy's early calls went unanswered. Goodness knows he was persistent. He was used to getting his way. He'd call my office every twenty minutes if he couldn't reach me on my cell phone. He'd insist that my assistant slip me a note or pull me out of a meeting. At first, I gave in out of pure fascination with the man. We were so different. I had gone to PS 158; he went to Andover. I like boxing; he liked golf. I'm a bleeding-heart liberal. He was quite the conservative.

We started to spend more time with each other over the second half of that summer, in 2007, once I had moved into the Surrey. Ours was not a perfect love story. It was an improbable one. When I first met Teddy I could not imagine ever being involved with someone like him. Not only because of his age, but also because he was so utterly different from me in every way. He was a Republican, a staunch one, who displayed in his home framed photos of himself with both George Bush Senior *and* Junior. I am a Democrat, one whose libido was curtailed by having to look at such pictures, and I told him so. He removed them. He was also a faithful, churchgoing Catholic, and when I say churchgoing, I mean he never, *not ever*, missed a Sunday Mass; not when we were sailing in the Caribbean and not when we went to Mumbai. In fact, even when he was in the Hamptons, he would arrange his return to the city based on whether he intended to attend church on Long Island or in Manhattan. Because his helicopter couldn't land in Southampton after sunset to pick him up, he'd have to plan on leaving in time to make Mass in the city. This meant missing a considerable part of his Sunday at the beach. But he did it and without grumbling. I, by contrast, was a pretty secular Hindu, going to my local temple in Queens mostly on major holidays. Though after the temple installed a canteen in the basement, my family noticed a considerable spike in my piousness (they serve the best masala *dosas* this side of Chennai).

Teddy was from another time, chivalrous to a fault. He was very mindful of respecting boundaries and never strayed from the principles he lived by. In the beginning, after that trip to L.A. on his plane, we didn't really *date*. We had dinner a few times, often with his sons, and he always picked me up and dropped me off at my hotel's front door. My husband had never picked me up; we always met at the restaurant or event. The only time we arrived somewhere together was when we had left the house together and shared the taxi, which I usually hailed for us on our corner.

But even beyond politics and religion there was a comically large list of differences between us. Teddy was not adventurous with food by any means. He hated spicy food, preferred fried chicken to chicken curry, enjoyed steak and pot de crème, not tacos and falafel. He liked country music. He was very athletic, playing golf with Vijay Singh and tennis with the Bryan brothers regularly. I only became sporty at thirty, when my vanity kicked in and I took up boxing to stay fit.

But Teddy and I connected emotionally, to both of our surprise. "I know what it's like to be on the outside looking in, Junior," he said once. He had always felt like a loner, and excelled at compartmentalizing the disparate elements of his life. He had traveled so far spiritually from his early life in Connecticut, and all he had been through in the intervening years—more time than I'd been alive—gave him empathy for where I was now. He was the most confident man I had ever met, and yet he confessed that there had been times when, before a big gamble, he'd been as afraid as a little boy.

Teddy was old-fashioned in almost every way. Even though I had sought out a divorce months before we'd met, that first summer, when I'd visit him at his home in the Hamptons, he'd insist on accommodating me in a guest room. This charmed me to no end. *Finally*, I thought, *a man who gives me some space!* But his adherence to decorum could also perplex me. Just before I moved into the Surrey, Dr. Seckin performed another endo-related surgery on me. Teddy was considerably worried for my well-being, laid up as I was, alone again in that big house. He sent a bushel of flowers but refused to come visit me because, he said, "It isn't right to enter another man's house, even if we're only friends. I know what my intentions are in my heart. And I don't belong there."

I had never met a man like him before.

Teddy was so well read, though wore it lightly and by the end of summer had devoured several tomes on Churchill and Gandhi, the history of India and its independence. He was a history buff, and he relished spouting obscure facts about Indian history at the dinner table both to check my own knowledge and to irk me. But deep down, this seduced me, too. I was touched that someone as busy as he was would voluntarily take serious free time to learn about my culture. Even with all his responsibilities at work (which included managing four companies, not only IMG), and his dedication to his boys, he somehow made ample time to woo me and make me feel he was always there for me. I didn't know where he got his energy. But while I was unbelievably lucky to have the full beam of his love shine on my life, I was also intimidated and overwhelmed by it. I had just come from a situation where I felt I wasn't meeting someone's expectations of me, and I knew agreeing to be the partner or girlfriend of a man like Teddy came with similar requirements. In spite of all the wooing, I was strangely despondent. I wasn't ready for Teddy. I couldn't understand why such a person, or any person, could be that kind, that patient, without wanting anything in return from me except my happiness.

So whenever we began to get too close, I came up with a reason to back off. He was too old for me, too unlike me, too pushy. But every time I'd tell him I couldn't see him anymore, I found myself missing his counsel, his knowledge, his wicked sense of humor. I missed his presence. I had to exert effort not to call him. For a time, my practical side won out. Fortunately, he was Teddy and he found ways to get his message across. He'd call my girlfriends and pull *them* out of meetings. His gumption makes me laugh now.

I was, in my way, seeking mentorship from Teddy, too, pumping him for advice while I started my jewelry business and began to build Easy Exotic spices and teas. Even though I was unsure I could be with him long-term, I thought that through our friendship he would impart to me a practical kind of entrepreneurial wisdom. But I was so naïve there, too. What Teddy wound up schooling me in was not business acumen, although he did indulge my every question and help me develop that aspect of myself. Teddy taught me about kindness, about love that is unconditional; a sentiment not dependent on acceptance, approval, or the expectation of something in return. It was the first time I would ever feel this from a man who wasn't my grandfather. And I didn't know what to do with it at all. If only I'd embraced our differences sooner. I didn't know it then, but we had so little time left.

chapter 10

He called me "Junior." Occasionally, he called me "Madam" when he wanted to make me the bad cop—as in "I'd be happy to join you at the Red Sox game, but Madam will never go for that." But he used "Junior" the most, his way of poking fun not just at our vast age difference, but also at my fixation on it. I called him "Duke."

We came up with his nickname on a trip we took to India in the spring of 2008. Teddy had never been to India. Four times before we met, he had planned to travel there on business, had even received the requisite immunizations, only to cancel his plans at the last minute. India seemed a world away to him and I could tell the whole idea made him tired. But I also knew the country and its history fascinated him. He felt that to fully realize his goals of expanding his company's interests, he would surely need to confront India at some point. Having me in tow to be a guide of sorts made the trip more surmountable. A few of his employees even took bets on whether he'd make it there. (Tom Ritz lost money, but was pleased for us.)

We were going to be staying in Jaipur, Rajasthan, at the Taj Rambagh

Palace, once the residence of the maharajah of Jaipur, which his family now operated as a lavish hotel. Before Teddy made the reservation, I had told him to not give them my real name. I often used an alias to check into hotels, to avoid unwanted attention. To keep the ruse simple, I always used the same name, which was—as a nod to my family, who might need to find me—my uncle's surname, Nathan. My full alias was "Dr. P. Nathan." Teddy thought this was hilarious. "What, you're a Jewish orthopedist now?" he joked the first time he heard it, then gleefully set out to come up with his own nom de hotel.

I rejected out of hand his first suggestion, Pee Wee Reese, the name of one of his favorite baseball players. "A real star," he said, smirking, "in the forties and fifties." (Again, because he knew it bugged me, he took great pleasure in underscoring his age.) The point, I reminded him, was to be *inconspicuous*. "Pee Wee Reese" was anything but. So he chose the name of another player, Duke Snider, a name recognizable to fans, maybe, but sufficiently unobtrusive for our jaunt in South Asia.

On our last night at the hotel, we returned to our room to a letter bearing the royal seal. Teddy opened it. It was from the grandson of the maharajah, who ran the hotel. His grandfather, he wrote, had been a Brooklyn Dodgers fanatic and would have been honored to know Duke Snider was staying at his residence. Teddy loved this letter. When we got home, he had it framed and hung it in his office next to Mandela's tin plate.

And so, we were Duke and Junior. We made an odd pair. As I said, we didn't pray to the same god or like the same foods. Let me tell you, though, of the two, our Hindu-Catholic union was nowhere near as troublesome for me as our gastronomic mismatch. For such a worldly man, his tastes were shockingly pedestrian. When we were together in India, he subsisted almost exclusively on scrambled eggs, toast, and club sandwiches with ketchup. In fact, everywhere we went, he ate club sandwiches. I teased him that he was single-handedly responsible for the club sandwich's omnipresence on room-service menus throughout the world. He loved steak and Italian food, especially when we were eating at stalwart Manhattan restaurants like Sistina, Elio's, and Il Mulino, where the waiters wore ties, the customers were important, and the portions were large.

What made his culinary limitations even more fascinating to me was that they existed despite his ability to eat anything anywhere he damn well pleased. Someone of his means could fly to Tokyo on a Monday just to eat *uni* and *o-toro* at Sukiyabashi Jiro. He could lunch the next day at L'Arpège in Paris, then pop over to Catalonia to grab a late dinner at elBulli. But for Teddy, the height of culinary achievement was a dry-aged rib eye. While I've been known to ramble on about "succulent" this and "glistening" that, the highest compliment he could pay any food was "Now, that's a good-looking steak."

At first, his stubbornness frustrated me. I wanted to share my love of food, my conviction that food could be—no, *was*—an adventure, with him. But I grew to love that about him. He made no pretense about his food preferences. And when you hang around ramen obsessives and fried chicken fanatics, as I happily do, someone who has no great interest in food can actually be a refreshing presence, a reminder of how much else there is to experience. As he'd gently chide me, "I know Picasso, you know pasta."

Part of the fun we had was catering to each other's desires, though he was both a better caterer and a better sport. Sure, I didn't gripe when Teddy flew in for dinner while I was filming *Top Chef* Chicago and insisted on dining at Gibsons, even though I was already gorged and distended. The steakhouse seemed to specialize in Flintstones-sized portions. His rib eye looked like it clocked in at just under five pounds. Even my Caesar salad came in what appeared to be a small rowboat.

Teddy, however, did a lot more than "not gripe" when I got an itch to try somewhere or something new. In the fall of 2009, for no particular reason at all—not my birthday, not Valentine's Day—he told me he wanted to take me on a fantasy food tour. You choose the restaurants, he said, I'll get you there. I named the two most exciting places in the world. He told me to pack my bags. Our first stop was to be elBulli. A week or two before the meal, Ferran Adrià, the chef of elBulli, very kindly e-mailed to ask if we had any allergies. Thank you for asking, I wrote, before I began my lengthy catalog of Teddy's aversions: olives, oysters, chilies . . .

Destination number two was Noma, the legendary Copenhagen restaurant. The food at Noma was Teddy's worst nightmare, whereas I couldn't have been more excited to try René Redzepi's pioneering neo-Nordic cuisine. I'd read all about the young phenom's fetish for foraging, for resurrecting ingredients once eaten but long forgotten, like tree bark, moss, and ants. Redzepi was famous for using almost exclusively products found or produced in the Nordic region: sea buckthorn, cloudberries, wild sorrel. His dishes reveal the arbitrary nature of our food system. We eat such a small portion of what's edible. Most of us pay dearly for prewashed arugula, even as we trample (edible, delicious) dandelions on the way home. To eat at Noma is to be transported to a very particular place, away from the world in which food travels thousands of miles before it reaches you, the world in which, no matter your location, you always have access to tomatoes, lemons, and cumin. Each dish at Noma disorients, gloriously: the ingredients provide a window into the past, while the presentation and techniques abut the future. To Teddy, the restaurant was nonsense.

His proof came with the first course. Seated at our blond wood table, adorned with the usual stemware, plates, and a vase filled with a few red flowers, we watched as our waiter arrived empty-handed. With a smile, he told us that our first course had already arrived. "Where?" we said as we stared down at the empty plates in front of us. "Right here," he said, gesturing at the vase. The flowers in it were nasturtiums, delicate and sweet with a nose-tickling radish-like bite. And tucked inside each one was a surprise: an edible snail. What I had thought were decorative sticks were actually malt bread.

I thrilled at the playful trick. In such a beautiful restaurant, I felt the desire to fully experience it, to revel in every moment, every sight and sound. Now I was told that I could experience a small part of this beauty through the most intimate act: eating it. Teddy's response was classic Teddy: "The best restaurant in the world and they're serving me a flower? I have hydrangeas in my garden that look more delicious than this." Not only was I asking him to eat a flower and a slug, but he was also paying through the nose for the pleasure.

When the next course arrived, Teddy looked down at the ice-filled mason jar set in front of us. It held two shrimp, each one about the size of my pinkie. "Okay, Junior, what are we eating?" he asked. I told him what the waiter had told me: we were supposed to dip the shrimp in the emulsified brown butter provided, then pop them whole into our mouths. Oh, and did I mention the shrimp were still alive?

"No way I'm eating mine," he said, "he's too cute," disguising his disgust with empathy. I grabbed one. As I contemplated my task, it was complicated by the shrimp, which had started to move. Teddy picked up one of his, and soon it was moving, too. I had finally summoned the courage to eat mine when he decided that in their writhing, the two little guys resembled tennis players swinging tiny imaginary rackets. When he dubbed them Rafael and Roger, I put mine down for good.

I couldn't have had a better companion for this meal than Teddy— not despite his teasing, but because of it. Meals like this are part cooking, part performance art. They toe the line between the sublime and the absurd, between decadence and debauchery. On which side of that line they ultimately fall depends on the chef, but also on the diner. Teddy kept me grounded. He reminded me that while this was swoon-worthy food that bordered on art, it was still just food.

Exaggerated derision figured prominently in our repartee. It was the way we coped with our differences. During the first hour of an afternoon spent watching golf, I'd groan, "How can you like this, Duke? It's just men in funny pants walking." Or I would gripe at the frequency with which he ate steak: "Well, I guess someone has to keep the cattle growers happy." But even as he made fun of my love for dishes featuring chickweed and white currants and bleak roe, he indulged it. He took great pleasure in seeing me happy. Never had I been courted so thoughtfully, thoroughly, and with such panache.

To see Teddy at Basement Bhangra was to understand the extent of his devotion. Basement Bhangra is a once-a-month dance party at a club in Manhattan (back then it was at S.O.B.'s) that at the time drew hordes of Punjabi grad students and other subcontinentally inclined dancers who grooved to North Indian music fused with hip-hop. The effect was a sort of cross between a high school dance and a disco hoedown. This was my happy place. To Teddy, who preferred Fleetwood Mac and Mozart and despised dancing, it was a hellscape. But nonetheless he came. And in the sea of young brown sweaty bodies, Teddy stood out like, well, like a sixty-eight-year-old white guy.

Because practically everyone in attendance at Basement Bhangra was Indian, I went resigned to being recognized. There were some stares and the occasional awkward conversation, each party straining to be heard above the bass. But the time I brought Teddy was different. People would approach me, and I'd prepare my cheery "Yes, I am Padma Lakshmi. Nice to meet you!" smile. "Is that who I think it is?" they'd ask, motioning toward my companion. "Is that really Teddy Forstmann?" These were MBA students, after all, far more interested in spotting the man who came out early against junk bonds than the woman best known for hosting a cable cooking show.

The closer I felt to Teddy, the stronger my practical side pushed back. Part of this was deeply buried guilt. The age difference between me and Salman had, I believed, played a major part in the undoing of our marriage. I had told Salman this and I believed it was true. Being with Teddy made me feel like a hypocrite. I could not help thinking about how Salman would feel when he heard the gossip. I felt ashamed, and very mixed-up.

For two years I told Teddy I didn't want a relationship, that I wasn't ready for one, and that even when I would be, I wasn't sure he'd be the appropriate choice—even as we spent more and more time together and grew closer and closer. Whenever something good happened, Teddy was the first person I called. Whenever I needed advice about work or to vent or was scared, I called Teddy. We were thick as thieves and intermittently lovers, and I somehow convinced myself that if I kept telling him I couldn't handle being in a committed relationship with him, I could keep us from getting too entangled romantically, yet preserve a friendship that was a main source of comfort and support at the time. But it was too late. We were already entangled. I just didn't want to accept it.

Part of me just wanted to play the field, honestly, as cruel as that is. For practically the first time in my adult life, I was single. Until that point, my romantic life had consisted of a series of serious, committed relationships, from my college boyfriend to Daniele to my husband. In the short time between my move back to the U.S. and the day I met Salman, I had briefly dated, but that was the extent of my life as a bachelorette. Now I had little desire to be anyone else's wife or main squeeze. I had had enough of smiling silently at all the fancy dinners, all the events that blurred into one another in a daze of cocktail dresses, champagne, cultured small talk, and hurt feelings at the end of the night.

All this "don't tread on my freedom" stuff was just catnip to Teddy. There was nothing he liked more than a challenge, and after a lifetime of being chased by women who wanted to pin him down, my loner vibe appealed to him immensely. And Teddy loved the idea of coming to someone's rescue. He had ample practice at it given his own personal history with his father, who suffered from alcoholism and other issues and often took out his frustrations on his mother. Teddy hated bullies and always rooted for the underdog. I had certainly filled his ears full of all my insecurities about making it without my husband and finding my own way. He could see I was scared, incredibly disillusioned about love, burned by bad experience, and wanting the world to go away. He would not go away.

Somewhat early in our push-pull, "come closer, now go away" routine, I met a man named Adam Dell. It was November 19, 2007, and I was on a book tour for my second cookbook, doing a signing at the Strand. It was also the day I would find a listing for what would become my first home. I remember using the folded sheet from the Realtor as my bookmark. A mutual friend of ours brought Adam to the signing and afterward we all went out to a small dinner thrown for me by my friend Luca. Later that night we went dancing, and I liked how dainty I felt in contrast to Adam's tall, broad-shouldered frame. I was with friends, letting loose after a horrendous year and a grueling book tour while at the tail end of a public divorce. It was therapeutic to dance and not talk. I felt liberated to a certain degree. He seemed to slip in easily among my friends and asked very little of me. There was a strong kinetic attraction between us. Nothing was verbalized or analyzed, but it was hanging in the air, daring me to do something about it. At that moment in time, just two months after my divorce, I didn't trust my feelings about anything, and indeed was anxious not to feel anything, really, for anyone.

Adam was about as different from Teddy, or Salman for that matter, as you can imagine. He was, for a start, my age. I hadn't been with someone my age since college. Adam was fun, liked Led Zeppelin and spicy food, and felt to me like the prom date I never had. He ignited a certain playfulness in me. I didn't know much about Adam, and I didn't really investigate because I felt I had enough on my plate as it was. Over the course of my book tour we kept in touch via occasional text. I didn't see him again until the following month in L.A., when I went to do an appearance on the *Ellen* show. Then I saw him once more a month after that, in mid-January, on his birthday. I had just returned from a New Year's holiday with Teddy. To commemorate my new life as a divorcée, Teddy had charmingly rented a beautiful boat named the *New Vida*. I was looking forward to the year ahead, hopeful and expectant.

So I kept seeing both men. My relationship with Adam illustrated to Teddy that I meant business about dating other people. But after a couple of weeks with Adam, I would miss Teddy terribly. I missed the verbal jousting, the wit, the all-consuming roller coaster that being with this charismatic man entailed. The whole thing was deeply unfair to Adam, because he never really stood a chance. No matter how easygoing and amenable he was to anything I threw his way, no matter how charming or thoughtful or fun, the fact was, my heart already belonged to Teddy, whether I wanted to admit it or not.

I would spend the better part of 2008 feeling that while it was exciting to have two such different men court me, I probably wouldn't wind up with either of them. I had very different experiences with each man. I rationalized that since I had been clear with both men about not wanting a serious relationship, and that I told them both I was dating other people, this made everything all right. That it was perfectly acceptable to date them both, even though I knew they both wanted more. I disregarded what I knew were serious feelings on both their parts. But beyond my own self-absorption, and my total lack of concern for whether I was hurting either Teddy or Adam, my feminist and willful side had kicked in. Why couldn't I date more than one man? Men did it all the time without compunction. While I had a right to my own freedom, I did not look too far into the future to consider the consequences of my actions. The heart wants what it wants, and it hears only what it wants to hear. Neither of the relationships I was juggling felt as casual to these men as I was treating them. And if I had stopped to investigate my own heart honestly, I would have seen that while I was utterly taken with Teddy, or occupied with Adam, I still sorely missed Salman. I didn't want to go back to my marriage, but the truth is that I wasn't over my ex-husband. I was rudderless and should have made myself be alone.

chapter 11

That same desire to take ownership of and forge a new life for myself, on my terms, had also been driving me to find a home I could call my own—a home *I* owned, a place that belonged solely to *me*, that wasn't contingent on a husband or a landlord. Freshly divorced, I had experienced a wound of displacement and homelessness moving into the Surrey that had just started to truly heal. I did not want to reopen it, ever. On a snowy day in January 2008, I unlocked the door to a home of my own, my first. The cute two-bedroom Alphabet City apartment on the fifth floor of an old brick tenement was a far cry from the Park Avenue townhouse I had spent the last few years in, but the place was all mine. I loved every inch of it.

The neighborhood was a vast change from the historically landmarked street on which my marital home stood. At that time, Alphabet City still had a lot of rats scurrying around car tires in the night. The sidewalk outside my building often gave off the faint stench of stale urine and vomit splattered there by the nightly young bar hoppers. But I loved the neighborhood's gothic weeping willows and scrappy communal gardens with their metal sculptures rusting under the heavy snow. And my little oasis was the quintessential image of what outsiders think a downtown New York apartment should look like. It had an open-plan kitchen with wooden cabinets I ripped the doors off and painted Moroccan red. The spare room had a load-bearing wall with two arches in the middle of it, but I made it work because I turned one half into my writing room and the other half into my dressing room. I made it as girly and feminine as humanly possible. My "ancient Egyptian" costumes from *The Ten Commandments*, along with various gowns and baubles I had been gifted over years of modeling, hung everywhere. It was wonderful just to have all my books and pictures back around me. Six months of being a gypsy and living in hotels and guest rooms had begun to wear me thin and jangle my nerves. I relished having my own space again, and the best part: I was finally in my own kitchen once more.

The first thing I did was unpack the pots and pans and cooking utensils. I wasn't really sure what to do with the half set of Tiffany's wedding china. But I was so giddy about being able to cook in my own kitchen again that I lost any of the rancor I'd had about the inevitable division of goods that is part and parcel of a marital breakup. I thoroughly savored going to Kalustyan's, my old standby gourmet ethnic store, and buying all my pantry ingredients. I lingered lovingly in their spice aisles like a bookworm in the stacks of an old library. I filled my basket with *ras el hanout, baharat, urfa* chili and sumac, green mango powder and *zaatar,* bottles of obscure hot sauces, *yuzu* and rose jam. I was in heaven. I went to Artisanal's cheese cave and splurged on everything that Chantal, my crusty French cheesemonger with a gravelly voice and perpetually smudged cobalt-blue eyeliner, made me taste: small putty-like wheels of goat cheese soaked in eau-de-vie and wrapped in grape leaves; a fluorescent wedge of mimolette, cracked and pungent and briny; and an oozing, stinky round of Camembert. I spent endless hours perusing the shelves of Pearl River Mart, picking out all manner of bowls, from large to tiny, from which I slurped everything from noodles to pasta to ice cream. I went to Patel Brothers supermarket in Jackson Heights, loading up on white turmeric and green mangoes and tindora, a small Asian squash that is my favorite vegetable. I replaced the many jars of oily Indian pickles I had had to leave behind when I became a hotel vagabond. I was reunited with the sublime mouthfeel of cold salted yogurt and rice spiced with crunchy fried mustard seeds, a dollop of various beloved pickles nestled into each bite.

I cannot remember the first complete meal I cooked in that kitchen in the East Village, although I know for a fact it must have contained a lot of aromatic *sambar* curry powder, because it was this taste, this remnant of home cooking, I longed for most in those last nomadic six months of misery. Teddy had been very generous with his living quarters. Upon coming home one afternoon and discovering me in his kitchen, he encouraged me to cook there whenever I wanted. He said no one other than his housekeeper had cooked him a midday meal in years, and the sight of me in an apron moved him almost as much as the indigestion he suffered later from the spicy lunch itself. After that I was careful not to pollute his tony Fifth Avenue penthouse with the odors of the subcontinent, even though his kids loved Indian food since they'd eaten it in South Africa.

But now I was home. In *my* home, *home* home, once and for all. I had had various apartments before in quite a few cities over the course of my life, but this was the first one I owned, and it felt good. A roof over my head and a place to be private, to cry, to laugh, to gorge, to hope, to dream, to wallow, and to pray for things was a salve to my soul. And cooking was indeed my salvation.

I made the staple chutneys and condiments I used regularly, like thick, pasty cranberry chutney with cayenne and fenugreek. I boiled carcasses in a heap of vegetables and aromatics for stock I could freeze. I spent whole weekends in the dead of winter filling tall canisters with lentils and pulses of every color. I bought black rice, red rice, brown rice, and of course basmati rice by the heavy jute sackful. I replenished my cupboards with all those rare and funky things I had discovered over my years of travel: dried black Omani limes and Szechwan peppercorns, kokum fruit skins and tins of glittering pieces of orange glacé. Some friends tried to remind me I was living alone and surely would not need all this. But they didn't get it. It comforted me to have all these twigs and leaves stuffed into my larder. On those new red shelves, I sought to replicate my grandmother's storeroom. I never wanted to leave the house again.

By my thirty-eighth birthday that September, I finally began to feel like I was getting my life fully back on track. I had settled into my new apartment. The show was doing really well. We had been nominated for an Emmy every single season since I had started, and though I in no way felt significantly responsible for this, it set me at ease about whether or not I truly belonged there. I had renegotiated a much better contract with the network, too, and I was beginning to take on other business ventures. I hadn't felt comfortable or confident about money since the height of my modeling days. And back then it had troubled me that my material security was based on my looks, which I neither had earned nor could count on in perpetuity. Now I made a living from my knowledge and skills and my efforts. I was self-reliant, and this feeling, this sense that I would indeed make it on my own, was crucial to restoring my faith in myself.

Somewhere in the middle of all the back-and-forth between *Top Chef* and Teddy and Adam that year, I had started to worry that I wouldn't get my act together in time to bear children. Despite my endometriosis, I hadn't given up on becoming a mother. And I now had enough money in the bank to splurge on freezing my eggs, something Dr. Seckin also vehemently encouraged me to do. But in order to do so, I was required to first undergo a battery of (expensive) hormone tests.

Seckin referred me to a fertility specialist, and as 2008 came to a close, I made the appointment. Early that winter, I dutifully took the tests. I was confident, or at least hopeful, while I awaited the results. When the fertility doctor called with my test results, I was making breakfast. I had just scrambled some eggs and delivered them to a crisp slice of sourdough, and drizzled the whole yummy thing with Tapatío Hot Sauce.

I sat on my couch, the plate perched on my knees, as the doctor leveled with me. The stress of my disease had taken a toll on my body. My ovaries, he told me with a typical medical professional's tact, were effectively even older than I was. Aging is hard enough on a superficial level. Your favorite features begin to wilt, like cilantro left out too long. The last thing you want to hear when you're staring down the barrel of forty is the discourteous surprise that your insides are even older. Still worse, he told me that it was highly unlikely I could conceive naturally—"the old-fashioned way," in his phrasing.

Fine, to hell with the old-fashioned way, what about in vitro fertilization? Even if we harvested my eggs, he said—after daily injections meant to pump my system into egg-laying overdrive before my ovaries officially threw in the towel—my chances were just 10 to 15 percent. By the time I hung up the phone, my scrambled eggs were cold. I picked up my breakfast and tried to take a bite. The toast, now damp, had lost its will under the pile of curds. The bread gave way, sending egg onto my sweatpants. The bits of curd looked like vomit, the hot sauce and egg and toast seeping their moisture into my sweatpants and the velvet couch. And vomiting was just what I felt like doing. I had squandered the best years of my life following Salman around the globe, going to amazing parties and grand literary dinners where he held court, but I had not tended to those parts of my womanhood that needed the most care. I knew something had been wrong and I had just pushed it away repeatedly while time marched on. I imagined my insides like those eggs; what I had once thought of as so healthy, full of vitality and life, now seemed to be a useless, deflated mess.

My desire to be a mother had played a significant part in the excruciating decision to end my marriage. I couldn't imagine introducing a child into our volatile relationship, so I had to end it and move on. Now I wondered: Had I left a man who, despite all his faults, truly loved me, just to chase a fantasy? Would I end up both childless *and* alone? The fact that I had two men in my life but had trouble fully committing to either one of them did not help matters. I had just come back from a Christmas trip to India with Adam and decided that while our holiday had been enjoyable, we didn't have enough between us to sustain the relationship. I just wasn't engaged enough mentally or emotionally.

I called Seckin to tell him what the fertility specialist said. I began to choke on my own cursing words as big, fat, rolling drops of salty water tumbled down from my eyes. I felt so stupid for not getting to the bottom of what I knew was wrong all those years. I couldn't help it. Had I not valued myself enough to investigate all of the signs month after month, year after year? Rage and self-pity swirled in my stomach at the thought of being barren.

I thought about how, during my first surgery with Dr. Seckin in 2006, he had made the grim discovery that I was missing part of an ovary. It had been removed by a previous doctor who, I suppose, had decided to keep the news of the collateral damage to himself. When I had come to after my fourth (or was it my fifth?) surgery just that past May of 2008, Dr. Seckin told me gently that he'd had to remove my right fallopian tube. He had prepared me for this possibility. Still, it stung. I was thirty-seven, with half of my equipment gone. Had I found Seckin earlier, I could have saved my left ovary, I could have kept my right fallopian tube, and I may have even been able to salvage my marriage.

Several weeks later, during a brutal New York winter, I walked to yet another doctor's office, past leafless trees that sent their spindly branches toward the sky. This meeting was to set a plan in preparation for harvesting eggs once my body was primed. In the early spring, after three months of vitamin supplements, hormones injections, and blood tests, and many thousands of dollars in bills, the doctor harvested three eggs. Today, I still think about them, frozen, occupying space in Midtown Manhattan, in a room behind one of those thousands of windows you think nothing of as you walk past.

I froze my eggs, something every woman who has the means to should do by thirty if she hasn't had children and has the faintest interest in being a parent. Just as insurance. I wished someone had told *me* that a decade earlier. I got three little eggs. But a few years earlier I might have gotten much more with the same effort.

My gratitude for finding Seckin remained, but I began to be angry that I hadn't had treatment earlier. I was outraged that in spite of all the best health insurance and access to medical care on both U.S. coasts as well as in London, I had been undiagnosed and misdiagnosed until well into my mid-thirties. And now, with half my left ovary missing and a right fallopian tube gone, I started to confront the fact that all this could have been avoided. Neela's daughter, my young cousin Akshara, always creative and articulate and brash, began to have problems with her periods. On trips to India, I saw her suffer, and her whole mood would change. I remembered being rushed to Mount Sinai and having gastric surgery to treat the symptoms when I should have been there to treat the cause. If I had known at eighteen, at twenty-two, or twenty-six, or even thirty, what was going on, I could have much more easily ensured my ability to have children; I could have had a hand in my own destiny, rather than expect it to miraculously be what the world told me it should. We take so much for granted, most of all ourselves.

In my mother's generation, if things got really bad, they'd just give you a hysterectomy. In fact, endometriosis is the number one reason women get hysterectomies. But now we have the technology and research to treat the illness. While there is no cure, there is ample treatment. And now that I was on the other side of that pain, I could see how much the disease had stained the very fabric of my life. I had missed a week out of every month because of pain that drove me to my bed, with painkillers and heating pads. I had effectively forfeited 25 percent of my life to this malaise! I was so angry that I would never get all that time back, all those missed opportunities, all the events of my life I had to sit out of, barred by my own body.

I did not want the next generation of women to go through what I, and millions of women, went through every month. I could see how significantly my life would have been different if I had had treatment in my early twenties, instead of at thirty-six. I thought of Akshara and her sister just beginning their adult lives. I had not been saved from the dread of my period those twenty-three years, but perhaps if I warned these young girls, they could be saved from what I went through. If we could get the word out, maybe this generation of mothers would not tell their daughters what ours told us, what they had been told by their mothers. This is not our lot in life. It doesn't have to be. There are so many things in this world that aren't treatable, but this disease certainly is. Pain, after all, is your body's way of telling you something is wrong.

Seckin had been asking me intermittently to speak to a few young patients who were going through the same thing I had gone through. These women had been afraid to get the surgery, or just had been having a hard time for whatever reason because of endometriosis. It is a very isolating disease. He felt that if they could talk with a neutral person outside their family who had been through it, they would feel less alone. They could also see through my journey that there was hope and they could, perhaps, feel better.

Once, a young girl stopped me in Seckin's office as I walked out after an appointment. She was very excited, explaining what a die-hard fan of *Top Chef* she was. I could feel the remains of the K-Y Jelly from the vaginal sonogram I'd just had seeping into the crotch of my underwear. The girl quoted several of my quips from Judges' Table and listed her favorite episodes, many of which I had trouble remembering at that very awkward moment. It was the only time I could think of that I wasn't altogether pleased to accept a compliment on behalf of my show.

Seckin called later that evening to ask if I would get in touch with the same young girl. She had initially been helped by the pill, he said, but now needed surgery and was reluctant to go through with it. She had what seemed like a rather tenuous relationship with her mother, at least from what the doctor could tell by their behavior in his office during visits. Seckin thought that she would respond to my reaching out because she was such a fan.

He connected me with other patients a few times, informally and ad hoc, and it had proved therapeutic, helpful in some way. Seckin had already organized a small patients' support group and I met some of his other ex-patients who helped out. There were lawyers, financial professionals, women from many walks of life all suffering from the same disease and giving one another support and listening when no one else would. Seckin saw the effects of our efforts and was seized by the idea that we should cofound a formal organization dedicated to endometriosis research and education.

At first, I resisted. I didn't know anything about running a foundation and from what I could tell, the doc was always busy and his practice was overflowing, so I wasn't sure how we were going to pull it off. And, too, I felt that talking about endometriosis was frankly the most unsexy thing in the world, that it would seal the coffin on any appeal I had left in the world past forty. I was so conditioned into thinking, ever since those early modeling days in Spain, that if I drew the curtain back on such an uncomfortable and almost disgusting thing that had been happening to me all along, I would extinguish any interest or attraction the public had in me. It was embarrassing to even consider talking in print and onstage about my illness. And who would listen anyway? But I had seen how profoundly my life had changed since the surgeries: my pain, my discomfort, my moods, my ability to handle stress. My gratitude for Seckin's treatment made me want to talk to each of those patients in his office. Seckin had alleviated so much pain and suffering for me that I couldn't in good conscience say no to his foundation proposal. Still, he lobbied for a whole six months before I finally acquiesced.

And so, in April 2009 we launched the Endometriosis Foundation of America, with funds cobbled together largely from Seckin, along with a lot of goodwill. We formed a board mainly out of the most active members of his patients' group, and asked his wife to help out, too. He and I worked our Rolodexes to death and begged everyone we knew to help and buy tickets to a fund-raiser we were calling "the Blossom Ball," which we threw together in sixty days. It felt good to channel my anger toward a cause and turn my pain into something positive. I had to learn how to speak about my illness publicly, and the practice I'd had in the minicounseling sessions with Seckin's other patients was not enough. But I learned quickly. I had no choice. To try to get the word out, we all thought I needed to tell my story with candor to one big news organization to garner support and interest in our mission. We needed to raise awareness so other women wouldn't have to go through what I had.

I asked my publicist and friend Christina if she could help spread the word about our new foundation. This was much different from the usual press junkets of talk shows and magazine interviews she worked on for *Top Chef*, but she was happy to try. I started telling her all about it and she helped me hone my message and navigate how to tell a very personal and, quite frankly, squeamish story to strangers in a public forum. I practiced on the phone with her late into the night before our fund-raiser, and tried to subdue the considerable embarrassment I felt about, well . . . talking about my vagina.

I agreed to an interview with *Newsweek*. I had already been on their cover and felt they would treat the interview fairly and respectfully. The first Blossom Ball was a success, mostly because we shanghaied our friends and colleagues into helping. Whoopi Goldberg, who, it turned out, was a sufferer, agreed to speak at the last minute and Fareed Zakaria agreed to MC. I was very nervous about speaking about such private things to a journalist. I had been burned so much, especially as it related to my private life, that I felt very shaky about the whole thing. But I kept thinking of my young cousin. I kept thinking of all the young girls I passed in the street, knowing that 10 percent of them were walking around feeling like I did every month for years and years. I thought of the women who lived in the public housing near my place downtown who probably didn't have the health insurance I had, or the regular check-ups, how they could afford even less than I could to miss all those days of work. I thought of my mother on her heating pad, how a doctor had removed her appendix. I thought of the rejection on my ex-husband's face and his utter lack of understanding or empathy or even belief that I was actually in the pain I said I was in.

After the Blossom Ball, I went off to film in Las Vegas. Teddy flew in weekly for overnight visits. I had abandoned the use of any birth control as unnecessary. I was in a very bad mood for most of the filming in Vegas that season. I'm sure the residual hormones used for harvesting my eggs had something to do with it. It was tiring and the arid and airless atmosphere of Vegas left me dry of any enthusiasm. I had also decided to quit smoking once and for all, galvanized by self-loathing for not tending to my own body. I was disgusted with all the habits of my past.

Ironically, Las Vegas is the only place you can smoke everywhere and anywhere you want. I had had enough and the clouds of smoke I was forced to walk through on my way to my room only reminded me of my own tacit and slowly self-destructive past. It was surprisingly easy to quit. I had quit once before, when Salman and I were first living together, because of his asthma. Then when he was not around I picked it up again. I could worry about his health but somehow not about my own. We throw ourselves away a little each day.

Dr. Seckin and I continued working diligently to set up the foundation after I completed filming the Las Vegas season. I was triumphant from quitting smoking and determined not to fall off the wagon again. Back in New York, my spirits lifted, I briefly saw both Adam and Teddy in the same week in June 2009. Overall, I felt a little like Wonder Woman. Invincible. It was a period of productivity and creativeness and also a new-found general optimism. I hadn't felt like this for several years.

That same spring, buoyed by the energy of helping to launch the EFA and finding my voice, I also managed to somehow launch an entirely new venture: a fine jewelry collection at Bergdorf Goodman. I had been designing jewelry for personal use for years, and was itching to do it more professionally. Many years earlier, as a favor to a friend, I had agreed to meet a young jewelry designer named Tara Famiglietti. A willowy slip of a girl, with fine blonde hair hanging loose around her high, prominent cheekbones, Tara has the biggest, bluest eyes I have ever seen. While she is staggeringly beautiful, at the time she had a sadness in her expression that moved me deeply. When she first showed up at my door with some of her samples, she looked cool and casually chic in that way that girls in Paris and London do. Soon after that first meeting, we became fast friends. I very quickly learned that her father, with whom she had been quite close, had just passed. She was also having a bit of man trouble. Tara and I found it very easy to confide in each other. I have always had very tight, long-lasting friendships with women, and often these women have been instrumental in my life. I sensed I could be that kind of friend for her at that time.

I began commissioning custom jewelry from Tara, starting with pieces for my wedding—modern interpretations of traditional Indian jewelry. I would also come to wear many of her delicate creations on the red carpet. Later, when I started filming the next season of *Top Chef*, I realized that many pieces in my own jewelry collection weren't right for what I was doing on TV. I wanted to design a capsule collection for personal use that would better fit my new role as host. I didn't much like what I was finding in my closet or in the shops. I wanted pieces that adorned the body, highlighted the nape of the neck or the small of the back, pieces that had movement and light but didn't upstage me, make too much noise at Judges' Table, or look inappropriate in the kitchen. I knew Tara was the only person to translate my vision.

My rapport with Tara is not only emotional or sisterly, it is also similar to the relationship many women in India have with trusted jewelers and artisans who come to the house to collaborate on family pieces. Whenever a member of our family had a jewel to be made or a stone to be set or reset (because someone had died and left the stone or there was an impending wedding and we needed to round out someone's trousseau), we called our family jeweler, Mr. Mani, from Kerala Jewellers. He had a slight tremor in his hands, and dark chocolate skin the texture of time-worn leather. He wore his white hair back-combed and Brylcreemed, and was always dressed in plaid *lungis* (men's sarongs). His magical toolbox fascinated me. Wooden with a complex hinge, it unfolded into a minidesk at which he sat on our veranda. His box was not unlike my grandparents' Godrej, containing secrets and drawers I longed to pull open. I loved watching him work meticulously with all his tiny tools and files. He would first sketch a simple pencil drawing based on my grandmother's descriptions of what she wanted a given piece to look like. Mr. Mani worked quietly and methodically, never flinching as my grandmother insisted he had misinterpreted her extremely precise directions. Jewelry signifies so much more than self-adornment in Indian culture. The pieces serve as personal talismans, and the women in my family take the subject as seriously as they do their cooking or how they fold their saris. I loved Tara's hand, and the way she interpreted and executed what was in my head so deftly. It felt like she had the same intuition Mr. Mani had had. The pieces Tara created for me to wear on *Top Chef* looked nothing like what she designed for her own line, but were something new and different; something immediately mine. We had an amazing shorthand between us, and often we finished each other's sentences.

Frank Bruni of *The New York Times* had spent several column inches in the paper dissing my sartorial choices when reviewing my first season on *Top Chef*. It had seemed unnecessarily cruel to me at the time and it still stung several seasons later. I am sure his slight was part of the impetus for my calling on Tara to design my accessories with me. It frustrated me that, as a woman, I had so much more attention focused on how I looked than, say, Tom, our head judge, did. But in hindsight, perhaps Bruni did me a favor. Whatever the origin, I *loved* making jewelry.

Bruni was not the first person to skewer me in the *Times,* though. No, Guy Trebay had that honor when he mused in the Style section on the reason for my appearances at the Bryant Park fashion shows, deriding me as a "brand-name goddess" and "semi-celebrated hustler," and failing of course to mention what I had told him: that I was there for the same reason he was, to report on the clothes for *Harper's Bazaar* in my style column. That article came out long before I started filming *Top Chef,* but it was from that point forward that I started to really struggle with developing a thick skin against media attention. Fortunately, as *Top Chef* progressed, most of the feedback from actual everyday viewers of the show was quite positive.

Plus, real professionals in the food world seemed increasingly to enjoy and appreciate the show.

Top Chef both made me happy and taught me much, but I was itching to do something creative in addition to my TV work, to explore other facets of my interests. A few random people had seen the pieces I wore and asked where to find them. Slowly, I also had girlfriends and other TV personalities ask whether they could borrow them. With a bit of money left over from my Pantene contract, I designed a small collection of samples to add to what I already wore on the show, with Tara as my technical hands.

Now emboldened but largely ignorant of how to run a business, I somehow thought we could start a company, basically out of my kitchen sink. At the time, I had a spunky and sweet assistant named Shayna, who was a talented photographer and wonderfully creative. She shot the samples for our look book and other materials, and we called the company the Padma Collection. The three of us worked together elbow to elbow out of my tiny writing room, until I rented out the place on the sixth floor above my apartment as an office. It was getting pretty cramped in my writing room with all our raw materials, molds, and computers; Tara's tools; and Shayna's camera equipment. The upstairs apartment served not only as an office, but as a beautiful showroom, too, and the big open kitchen it had was perfect for testing recipes. The showroom was also a good meeting place for the foundation's board, as up until then we'd been meeting in Seckin's waiting room.

With all that was going on, I got it into my head that we should have the new office blessed, as I had done for every place I had ever lived, *except* my marital home. My ex-husband was a staunch fundamentalist atheist and had no patience for worshipping God in any form. I am pretty secular but didn't mind hedging my bets. I called a couple of priests from my temple and they came in from Queens to bless our new space. They brought fresh mango leaves, coconuts, and various idols and camphor to burn during the *puja*.

My cousin Rajni and her husband came to the blessing, with their infant son, Sidhanth, dressed in traditional clothing, looking every bit the perfect little Brahmin boy, with the customary horizontal three lines of *vibhuti* smeared across his forehead. It was wonderful to see young, hipster Shayna sitting cross-legged next to the *veshtie*d priests as they chanted in Sanskrit on the rooftop of our Alphabet City digs. It was moving to share a deeper part of my own heritage with Tara, who had been one of the people who had quietly helped me pack up to move into the Surrey just two years earlier, when I was too weak from surgery to do so myself. I watched the smiling face of Michelle, my makeup artist, with pleasure as I bounced and held my nephew in my arms. Michelle had been and would be with me through so many seasons of *Top Chef,* by my side for the most challenging days, like in Las Vegas when I almost threw up on camera from the heat, crippling menstrual cramps, and too much food for one person to consume. She had patched up my streaming eyes when I could not stop crying behind the set's kitchen door, because of how much I still missed Salman.

Through the smoky haze of incense, I watched my cousin Rajni instinctively rise and bend to get whatever the priests needed at exactly the right moment, in a way that I could not, because I had left India before I could properly learn the technicalities of such rituals. She stepped in gracefully and silently and made everything so seamless as her sari rustled about her. Like Neela, Rajni had always been more of a sister to me. She has been there for almost every milestone of my life, observing and playing her part in the hierarchy of our family. Her life had been so different from mine. She and her husband, Ananth, whom we had all known since we were kids, had lived in the old neighborhood since childhood, until moving to the States as adults just a few years before. I could not help thinking about how differently my life might have turned out if my parents, like hers, had had a happy marriage. Who would I have become if my mother and I had never immigrated to the States? My work in food, fashion, and jewelry was definitely a result of all my travels, of the commingling of cultural influences I got to experience because I'd always had one foot in the East and one foot in the West. At that moment, I gave thanks for all the circumstances of my life that brought me there, to that very place in the East Village. I was happy in our treehouse workshop with friends, family, and worker bees around me.

It felt good to hear Sanskrit echo in that office. And it comforted me to bring the various aspects of my current life together with the deepest spiritual origins of where I had come from. Like many immigrants, I had always kept my Eastern and Western lives compartmentalized. Not since I had left the comfort of my home and marriage had I felt a cohesiveness of being, a joining of my two very real identities. In that moment, finally, my American self and my Indian self were totally at peace as one.

chapter 12

Those first six months of 2009 were so busy, so productive, that time seemed to move faster than usual, and so I didn't notice at first when my period was late. I could hardly keep track of what day it was already. Like so many women, I had spent my entire sexual life trying not to get pregnant. My mother had always reminded me of her exceptional fertility (she had only one child, but my conception had been on the first try). It could be hereditary, she'd warn me. Be careful. And so I had been. But that had been before the fertility specialist's frank appraisal of my reproductive equipment. And though his conclusion had devastated me, it had also freed me from the worry of using birth control. Small consolation, but some nonetheless. For the previous six months, I had been less careful than I'd been in the past—I had been pretty much told there was no way I could conceive, after all. At least, not "the old-fashioned way."

But I was late. And despite the endo, I had always been regular—like clockwork. Was it possible? Could I be pregnant? I called Dr. Seckin. He sighed, sweetly, and told me to come in for a sonogram. Lying there, my stomach coated in jelly, I stared at the screen showing a hazy image of my uterus. I watched him whack the side of the monitor with his palm, as you would an old TV. "See this area?" he said, pointing. "If you were pregnant, you'd see a black spot right here." I saw nothing. I joked that maybe I had a hysterical pregnancy. "Not hysterical," he said. "Wishful."

Another week and no period, yet strangely, I had many of its symptoms: I felt tired. I was ravenous. My boobs were sore and swollen. Confused, I called my friend Sharon, who had told me her early pregnancy symptoms mimicked those of her period. I thought about calling my mother, but worried that she'd be too emotional. I needed someone who could maintain a clinical reserve. So I called my aunt Premi, a psychiatrist, who urged me to get a blood test to be sure. I finally gave in and asked my mom about her pregnancy. "Paddy, I can't remember," she told me. "That was forty years ago!" Thanks for the reminder, Mom. I called Seckin's office again. He was away in Iceland at a conference. I filled in Kim from his office, who told me to come in for a blood test and added an excited "I'm so happy you're trying!" But I wasn't trying.

Several fretful days after the blood test, I got a call from a strange number. I was in a rush as usual—my hair sopping wet, late for an interview with *TV Guide* and afterward lunch with the editor in chief. I picked up the call. It was Seckin, calling from Iceland. "Padma, you must come here," he said, the bad reception thickening his charming Turkish accent. "It's like being on another planet!"

"Is that why you're calling?" I asked. "To tell me about Iceland?"

"Padma, I'm standing on a glacier, in the full glory of Mother Nature." I knew then. By this point, I had known Seckin for years. I was well acquainted with the genuine sense of amazement that medicine and the human body inspired in him, even after decades of practice. I knew he wouldn't tell me this news from inside his hotel room. He had wanted to be in a miraculous place when he told me of my own miracle.

Seckin forbade me from telling anyone yet. The risk of miscarriage, for all women in the very early stages of pregnancy, is higher than most of us realize, unnervingly so for women my age. And because miscarriage is often a private tragedy, few of us understand that seeing a plus sign on your EPT is not the end of the story that movies make it out to be.

I hung up the phone, still in a daze. I slipped on pants, made one last attempt to dry my hair, raced downstairs, and hailed a cab. In the quiet of the car, in what felt like the longest cab ride of my life, the news hit me at last. I couldn't stop smiling. Hearing doctors tell you that you can't get pregnant does not extinguish the hope. Only after months of wrestling with the idea had I been able to haul the news of my infertility from the abstract and into reality. I had just begun to accept it, to make plans that took it into account. Now that mental struggle abruptly ended. I was purely, simply happy.

I wanted so badly to tell someone, but I couldn't call anyone from the cab. Though I'm on TV, I can still walk the streets of New York more or less anonymously. Among cab drivers, however, many of whom are from the subcontinent, I'm frequently recognized. Highly personal conversations are a no-no. So I was especially thrilled that my friend Christina was joining me for the interview. I got out of the cab, took her aside, and whispered my news. I felt giddy at hearing the words come out of my mouth out loud. Christina's eyes got very wide and she beamed a smile from ear to ear. After the meeting, a question began to nag at my giddiness: not so much "How?" but the far more uncomfortable "Who?" This the tabloids would soon address with their usual delicacy.

I never announced my pregnancy. I started showing and the press figured it out in the way they often do, with absurd speculation that's wrong until it's not. Just after the Emmys in late September a New York tabloid ran the article: "She's Pregnant!" accompanied by a photo of me standing beside my cousin Manu on a red carpet with my hand resting near my belly. "And

That's the Father!" the headline read. Unaccustomed to brilliant tabloid guesswork, Manu was horrified.

After the initial speculation the press wouldn't stop harping on the fact that I hadn't revealed the name of the father of my child. This prying and scrutinizing of my personal life in the pages of the tabloids was beyond anything I had previously experienced. The truth was that I didn't know the paternity myself, until late that September. That early fall I was feeling pretty shaky. Guilt and the shame of how I had not only hurt Teddy and Adam but had also effectively embarrassed my whole extended family swirled around in my head, mixing with the undeniable joy and elation that I would, incredibly, be a mother after all. My emotions blew hot and cold simultaneously, and I could not tell what was due to my fluctuating hormones, and what was due to the very real and complicated facts of my life, induced by my own cavalier insistence on doing whatever I wanted.

Even though my doubts about my future with Teddy lingered, I found myself wishing desperately that he was the father. The fact of this should've told me all I needed to know about my feelings for him. But before I could take that line of thought any further, I had to tell him my news: my miracle in one breath, an uncomfortable truth in the next. I told him about two weeks after I found out. He had been in London with his sons and my cousin Manu, who had by this time finished law school and started working with Teddy.

Teddy had wanted us to have a baby together. We had even discussed the idea months before, when I had my first egg frozen. "Why don't we just inseminate those eggs and get on with it?" he asked. My answer then was the same as when he'd suggested we get married the year before: "Let's wait a little and see." This became a refrain for me. Teddy, always decisive, would counter, "I don't exactly have time to waste. Do you?"

Now I would tell him that against all odds I was pregnant and that there was a good chance the baby wasn't his. We had been open about everything. He knew every doubt I had about our relationship. He knew I was at times seeing someone else. Still, none of this would cushion the blow. Because for there to be doubt about the paternity, I had to have been with both men within a week or two. Who wouldn't be hurt to hear that?

When I told Teddy, I had to quickly follow the good news with the excruciatingly bad news. He was, understandably, very, very angry. I saw his face go white, and then beet red. He started to pace vigorously in the small living room of my apartment. It was as if the room could not contain him, or as if his body could not contain his fury at the information he had just received. He yelled for some time, the first and only time he had ever spoken harshly to me, hurling insults my way. He did not say he would leave me, but he wanted no part of any scenario that included Adam. He had been aware of Adam, and while I saved him the details, I had been quite frank with him all along. I think he assumed my dalliance with Adam was something I had to get out of my system, or would grow out or tire of. He was enraged. He wanted to punch something, he said, but didn't know where to turn. He needed to leave my home to blow off the steam that was quickly rising, but I wouldn't let him out of the house for fear of what trouble he would get into.

Hot, heavy tears rolled down my swollen cheeks as I barred the elevator door with my body. In that moment, the sudden rush of how badly I had squandered the love and kindness this man had shown me began to sink in. I had no choice but to bear the full brunt of the consequences of my actions. I had to help Teddy express and expel the utter disgust he felt for me and the situation. I did everything I could to keep him in my home. I didn't want him to have to deal with this alone or with anyone else. What would they say to him anyway? "I told you so"; "That girl is trouble"; "Get as far away from that mess as soon as possible"?

Teddy did not waver from what he believed, even in that bind. When I said that I didn't know what to do yet and had to sort things out, he jumped at me without blinking. "The only thing, Padma, that would be worse than this, that I will never forgive you for, is not keeping this baby. I will never speak to you again if that happens." This caught me off guard, even though I knew full well about his feelings on the subject of abortion and a woman's right to choose. It was certainly another issue we differed vehemently on, but I was startled by his aggressiveness and his assumption that that's what I would resort to: the easy way out. But who could blame him?

Sometimes we kid ourselves when we imagine our lives, expecting that everything will neatly fall into place. In my case, I had expected to meet someone who was "appropriate" and who I deemed a good match, fall in love with him, and then start a family with him before my biological clock stopped ticking. For whatever reason, Teddy had fallen into my life and would not leave. Adam had come into it, too, and kept reappearing, or I for some reason kept drawing him back to me. I had assumed a future with either man made no sense, little knowing how important a role each one would play in my life.

When I told Adam the news, he didn't know what to do. I had broken things off with him that past February and the hard truth was that we had not seen each other since, except for the moment we had fallen back together briefly in June. Adam had moved back to Texas and on with his life. I couldn't blame him.

Teddy had implored me not even to involve Adam, and was frustrated and angry when I did. Teddy had to overcome not only his own anger and pain, but also the embarrassment I had caused him publicly, which the press only magnified all over the world. The only thing that was missing from this emotionally nauseating picture was morning sickness, for which I was very glad indeed.

I respected Adam's wishes to be left out of things for a few weeks but could not contain myself any longer. I had grown up without knowing my real father. My grandfather and the rest of my family had, in their fury, ripped up every wedding photo that ever existed, and so I had no idea of what my father even looked like. For so much of my life, there had been huge gaps in the information about my lineage, a whole side of my genealogy that no one wanted to discuss. I remember going out to eat *chaat* with Neela as a child and looking around at all of the men who would be about my father's age. I wondered if any of them could be him. Did I look like him? I had always wondered how my life would have been had I known my father and felt wanted by him. I wanted *my* child to know exactly where she had come from and to know that she was very wanted indeed.

I didn't want my child to have the same identity crisis or hole in her sense of belonging as I did. I realized that asking one man to stay with me in spite of my carrying another's child, and asking another man to be involved with the child I was carrying even though I did not want to be with him, was expecting a lot. But I knew that this was the right path for me, and the baby, though I could not tell if I would be able to will this situation into existence.

I also thought it would haunt both Adam and me if we concealed the baby's true paternity. Adam had always expressed a strong desire to start a family. Both his brothers had several children, and he longed to have his own. Thinking about how hurt he must be about the fact that this was not how he had wanted to start a family and that it was out of his control, I could not blame him for reacting the way he did.

I spent many nights in my East Village apartment, tossing and turning in bed, unable to sleep. I had not wanted to hurt anyone, only to have some space and freedom without a commitment. But I had hurt two people immensely. I had tried very hard to restart my life on my own terms. I would never have planned on having a baby this way, but I was not sorry she was here, in my belly. I resolved to do everything for the good of this child. I knew I would have to face the full brunt of all the gossip and embarrassment, the awkwardness and complicated circumstances around this pregnancy. So be it. I would take my medicine now, as much as I could up front.

So, privately, Teddy took a paternity test. Teddy asked Dr. Seckin to tell him directly, so he didn't have to hear the news from me. He was worried about his reaction if it turned out he wasn't the father, and he wanted to be able to process the information without fear of upsetting me. The news was not in his favor.

Teddy got the results while I was in California for the Emmys. *Top Chef* was nominated again. I was in my suite at the Chateau Marmont, feeling tired as I looked down from my balcony at all the Hollywood revelers in the garden below. The days before the Emmys are a marathon of luncheons and parties. My feet were hurting and I had no enthusiasm for joining in the festivities. I just wanted to know if Teddy was the father of my child. I went back into my room and dialed Dr. Seckin's cell phone. Low and heavy, Seckin's voice when he said my name told me everything I needed to hear. The sound of a woman laughing filtered in from the garden.

I returned to New York that following Monday. In a moment of great sadness and disappointment, Teddy implored me to keep the results between us. He would raise her as his own, he said, whether he and I ended up together or not. But I couldn't subject my child to that fate, nor could I do that to Adam, however I felt about him. Teddy was broken when I refused. I thought I'd lost him then. Now I needed to tell Adam. His initial reaction just to the news of my pregnancy had not exactly been happy. I dreaded telling him and kept procrastinating. Finally, weeks later, in November when I could stand it no longer, I insisted he visit me in person, so I could let him know he was the father.

Up until very late in the pregnancy, we couldn't agree on what we would do. How involved would Adam be in the baby's life? He had always wanted to be a dad, but he did not at all look forward to being a dad to a child who had her own family. We spent hours on the phone, trying to talk through the different scenarios. I wanted an option where I stayed with Teddy, but Adam would still be a part of the baby's life and our child would know she was loved by everyone. I didn't want to lie about who her father was. I also didn't want to lose Teddy. I had finally realized the high caliber of the man I had before me. I now had to set about making sure I did what was best for the baby, while also making sure Teddy understood how grateful I was that he had stayed by my side. I did not take that second chance lightly.

Sometime in early December, Teddy went with me to get a sonogram. Generally I went either with my cousin Manu or with a girlfriend. This time, no one was free to accompany me. Usually I could feel the baby kick or move from side to side, but for a few days I felt no movement at all. I felt uneasy going alone. Teddy overheard me on the phone to Seckin saying I was very worried. I had been feeling uncomfortable and getting larger. I hung up and looked at him silently. He was reading the paper, and I could see him trying to figure out in his head whether he was ready for this. The moment seemed very long, with him pondering whether he could actually stomach it and me trying to summon up the courage to actually ask him out loud. I asked halfheartedly, sheepishly.

Teddy was woefully delinquent in attending his own yearly checkups. He hated doctors and any and all medical stuff. But he was a gentleman above all else, especially when it came to women. And he could rarely refuse helping someone in need. He acquiesced with the same enthusiasm with which one schedules a colonoscopy. His expression told me that for him, the only thing worse than going was not going.

He met me at Dr. Seckin's office, around the corner from his apartment on Fifth Avenue. It was awkward at first. He didn't know what to expect, and I didn't know what I could expect of him. Maybe he would just sit in the waiting room? When we got there, two or three other women were reading magazines in the waiting area. I was directed to a small examination room, and after a glimpse at the waiting room, every seat full with a woman waiting to see the doctor, he quickly followed me in. To Teddy the only fate worse than being confronted with all the gory details of my condition was being subjected to the curious eyes of all those hormonal women outside. This was the first time Teddy had seen the inside of a fully functioning gynecologist's office in all his seventy years. The office had been closed when he had his blood taken for the paternity test.

The exam room was very small, about seven by eight feet, and very brightly lit, too brightly lit. There was a small stool on wheels tucked to the left of the exam table and little floor space for anything else. I lay on the table and pulled my jeans down. I lifted up my sweater and scooched higher up on the table. I had been to these sonogram appointments so often that by now I just skipped the step of putting on the paper gown, to stay warmer in the room. The sound of the crumpling and tearing of the thin paper sheet underneath me seemed obnoxiously loud. Teddy shifted from one foot to the other, visibly uncomfortable. He didn't know where to stand. He didn't know where to look. To my left was the sonogram screen. Teddy stood next to it, leaning against the wall by the door. Perhaps he felt this was a safe place for him, since he would have to completely turn away from me to see into my womb on the screen. Teddy suffered from vertigo, and I knew that look, but now he was also suffering from claustrophobia. A tear rolled down my left temple along my hairline and into my ear. He gently grabbed my hand. His hand felt heavy, soft, warm, and large, with calluses at the base of his fingers from years of golf and tennis.

Seckin came in and Teddy stiffened. He'd gone from trying to reassure me back to stoicism in a flash. Good old Seckin understood the emotional subtleties of men accompanying women in my condition to his office. And of course, Seckin was fully aware of the delicate circumstances, too. He deftly handled Teddy's presence with wisdom, compassion, and grace. Seckin gently asked Teddy to move to the other side of the exam bed so he could reach the machine and the wand connected to it. Teddy obliged. This time I searched for Teddy's hand with my right hand. The cold jelly squirted onto my abdomen made a farting noise coming out of the bottle, breaking the tension in the room. Seckin laughed and said, "Sorry," then moved the sonogram screen, shifting it for better viewing from his and Teddy's perspective. My eyes were glued to the monitor, but I was also acutely aware of the weight of Teddy's hand in mine.

"There! Here we go," said Seckin.

Teddy had been looking down at his shoes, but now looked up at the screen. "What is that?" he asked.

"It's her heart," I answered. I squeezed his hand, and we both saw her tiny heart pulsing away on the screen, he for the first time.

"Alll gooood," Seckin pronounced in his singsong, Turkish lilt.

I was scared Teddy wouldn't be able to handle it. There was a good chance he could walk out of that examination room and out of my life forever. I was also worried that the growing existence of this child would continually be a reminder of how I had hurt him, and of the embarrassment my actions had caused him. Seeing the growing baby in my womb could make it all too real for him. It could have scared him away. Who could blame him? Why would he still want to be involved with this mixed-up woman who had caused him so much pain? Most men would have run the other way, but Teddy wasn't most men. And I suppose I, too, needed to know if he *was* going to stay or go, before the baby came. I had had no guarantees from Teddy up to that point, only a sincere promise to try to make the best of the very hard position I had put him in.

There we were, holding hands and looking at this new life willing herself into the universe through me. Once I saw that the baby was indeed okay, I couldn't take my eyes off Teddy. It did something to him, to witness her beating heart that day, in that little room. It did something to me, too, watching him witness it. In the reflected blue light of the sonogram screen I saw so many different emotions flicker across his face. Teddy always wore his feelings on his sleeve. He tried very hard to maintain a stiff upper lip, but I was pretty good at reading his eyes. I saw flashes of wonder, anger, deep pain, frustration, sadness, amazement, compassion, bittersweet longing, all of it. I wondered what he was thinking about. Was he angry with me? Did he feel insulted to even be there, doing another man's duty? Did he resent me? Did he feel unable to express it, as his sense of chivalry would not allow him to speak to a woman harshly, especially one who was pregnant? Did he regret the years gone by in his life when he was conquering the business world and not experiencing what his peers were at home? Was he upset that this was how he was now forced to experience a new life entering the world for the first time? Was he thinking about his own sons, and how he never got to experience this stage of their development? Did he still feel squeamish and out of sorts because of the setting? What would he do now? What did he feel now? Was he just being a good friend or did he still love me? Did he even know? I didn't know if the vision of that little heart beating away mightily on that screen would push him away or propel him toward me. Both were totally plausible outcomes.

All those emotions and feelings he may have had inexplicably somehow galvanized together into love, pure and simple. In that moment, he had decided to see the glass as more than half full. Whatever he saw tugged at his insides and at mine, too. He looked directly into my face for the first time that day and I could feel the warm sunshine of his love. It took my breath away. He smiled and pointed to the screen. "This is all we need to think about," he said. "This is all that matters." That little beating heart on the sonogram had stolen his heart, and in turn Teddy had stolen mine, for good.

In many moments, what Teddy taught me the most, through his actions, much more than any business strategy or financial acumen, was unconditional love: how to receive it and how to give it.

chapter 13

Despite the drama, the majority of my pregnancy was blissful. I had a very happy and healthy first trimester. I had no
morning sickness, luckily, and even though the baby was too small to do
anything, I imagined I could feel her fluttering in my tummy, almost like a
tadpole swimming inside my womb.

I loved the mellow buzz I felt being pregnant, like the tipsiness after a
first glass of champagne. I liked my body as it rounded. I felt sexy, voluptuous in a "She's a Brick House" way. I knew that pregnancy, along with
my fortieth birthday, less than a year away, would usher in a fundamental
shift in the trajectory of my breasts, arms, and thighs. This weight gain,
of course, was unlike my past fluctuations. I felt liberated from the normal worries about my figure. My body had a higher purpose. Putting on
pounds wasn't just inevitable but also necessary. So while I still had to
participate in the mental tug-of-war between what I wanted to eat and
what I should eat, the prize of winning was no longer a flat stomach—it
was a healthy baby. Vanity is a powerful force. For so long, beginning perhaps with that accidental audition at Spanish *Elle*, vanity had governed my
eating habits. My vanity never quite kept me from giving in to that bowl of

coconut cream curry or those couple of (okay, fine, several) pieces of fried chicken. But it made me feel guilty about the indulgences—guiltily guilty, because I'm aware enough to know that my guilt is unproductive. Now I ate for the baby, not for the reflection in the mirror.

In the early days of my pregnancy, I, like so many almost moms, subsisted on a steady diet of prenatal vitamins and "What the Heck Should I Eat Now?" books. The instructions were daunting, to say the least. The stakes were higher, too: no longer would my inevitable dietary lapses only reveal themselves in my butt or belly rolls; they could affect my child, too. Cooking dinner after a full day of work was hard enough without this added pressure. So I soon shelved those manuals. After all, every reliable author seemed to agree on the same strict regimen of common sense and moderation.

The extent of the moderation recommended by the books surprised me, though. According to the *Mayo Clinic Guide to a Healthy Pregnancy*, which became my pregnancy bible, mothers-to-be need to increase their calorie intake by only 150 to 200 calories per day in their first trimester—little more than an extra banana, a thin slice of bread with peanut butter, or a glass of milk. Whatever happened to "eating for two"?

As someone who had long fantasized about my next meal halfway through my current one, I was familiar with this challenge. Yet now instead of an "eat less of this bad-for-me food" strategy, by which one could theoretically stay slim, I adopted an "eat more of these good-for-me meals" policy, which would nourish the little person inside me. And since I was going to gain no matter what I ate, I finally got to eat as much as I wanted, so long as the food was nourishing.

Highly processed foods were out altogether. Fried chicken and its ilk would become "In Case of Emergency" fare. I doubled down on any favorites that required minimal fussing. I roasted summer corn over my stovetop's flame, channeling the street vendors in India who charred ears over charcoal near temple doors. Plenty of lemon, salt, and smoked paprika or mild chili powder added enough flavor that I never missed my typical pat of butter, which at times made me a bit queasy. I made huge salads, colorful collections of vegetables and herbs, which I kept exciting with an ever-changing array of condiments—essentially, some flavorful ingredient (sherry vinegar or mustard, *yuzu* or yogurt) that I'd turn into dressing with very good first-press olive oil. Perhaps the most dramatic change I made in my diet was the regular addition of red meat. Aside from the no-proteins-barred eating fugues of *Top Chef,* I didn't eat much beef, lamb, and the rest—a lingering habit from my vegetarian childhood. Yet now I did once a week, for the iron and calcium. I found myself relishing my weekly seared skirt steak and the task of coming up with new ways to sauce meatballs.

Some decisions weren't so straightforward. Most women renounce alcohol and caffeine. The jury is still out on whether small amounts of either one will affect your baby. Still, the choice to play it safe seems like an easy one to make—that is, until you're forced to make it. *Of course I'll give it up!* I thought, gliding on the winds of idealism that marked my early days of pregnancy. Next thing I knew, my eyelids would feel even heavier than my bloated body, and I'd be plodding to the corner for coffee. A tea drinker for most of my life, I switched allegiance for nine months. I did manage to stick to one cup a day. Alcohol was easier to quit, though after the first trimester, which is the riskiest time to drink, I enjoyed a small glass of wine or champagne now and again.

I was drawn to comforting foods, the foods of my childhood: soupy mixed vegetables stewed with ground fresh coconut and curry leaves, *kichidis* (dishes of spiced rice and lentils), and of course my beloved yogurt and rice dish, *thayir sadam.* Whatever I ate, I put in a deep bowl, so it was all the easier to eat with my feet up. I didn't have many ultra-specific cravings, except for cinnamon, which I mainly consumed in milky banana shakes, and, strangely enough, good old yellow mustard. When the urge struck, I was powerless. About six months into my pregnancy, it assaulted me on the way out of Bergdorf Goodman, where I had been attending a trunk show for the Padma Collection. My mouth watered at the thought of the sharp, vinegary taste, so I made a beeline across the street to Central Park and the nearest hot dog vendor. I had been very conscientious about avoiding processed foods, but that day those steamy little links floating in their murky New York water called out to me. This was going to be my one very bad transgression.

I ordered a dog piled with relish and sauerkraut, then drenched in yellow mustard. "More?" the vendor asked, incredulous, as I gestured at him to squirt on yet another stripe of mustard. I found the closest hilly patch of grass, plunked myself down, and devoured the thing in four bites. My only regret was that I hadn't ordered two, because I then had to stand up to get a second one. This was no easy task. For my appearance at Bergdorf, I had dressed in an attempt to look chic, in black leather and heels and gold chains and bracelets galore, though "chic" was becoming more and more difficult as I swelled. So when my several attempts to heave myself up failed, I ended up back on the ground, shiny legs and arms flailing, gold bands jangling—a Mr. T–like beetle stuck on its back.

For much of my pregnancy, I had continued to work out, and box, too, but Dr. Seckin forbade me to lift heavy weights or jump or skip rope. He ordered me to go to regular weekly sonograms and was extremely concerned with the prospect of miscarriage and the baby's health in general. He became a sort of Olympic coach who checked in with me almost daily. It had been a while since he had practiced obstetrics on a regular basis, but he was watching me like a hawk. He himself had not believed it possible for me to produce this pregnancy totally naturally, and until the baby was out safely, I could tell that he would not let me out of his sight. This was, after all, his professional miracle as much as my personal one.

One day in early October, somewhere in my second trimester, I went to my usual sonogram, and Seckin saw something he didn't like. He sent me to Lenox Hill Hospital for another sonogram and that doctor confirmed what he suspected. I had developed placenta previa. Previa is a condition that occurs when the baby's placenta partially or completely covers the opening of the cervix at the base or bottom of a woman's uterus. It's normally supposed to grow on the side or top of the uterus. The placenta provides all the nutrients to the baby as well as removes waste. The danger with previa is that a woman can bleed excessively before or during delivery because of the placenta's position. In any event, this was not good news at all, and provided another layer of worry for all of us.

I was immediately forbidden to do any exercise of any kind. Seckin informed me that many endo patients do suffer from previa, but that it often happens to mothers who've never had endometriosis as well. Figures I'd get this, too, I thought. Up until this time, I had felt a bit of general fatigue, but I had also experienced a low-level hormonal high pretty much constantly since getting knocked up. I was a pretty happy pregnant lady. Seckin forbade me to exert myself in any way. Seckin is a very excitable type, who gets pretty emotional, especially for a doctor who is supposed to be calm in the face of his patients' anxiety. But all that bedside manner went out the window, it seemed, when it came to me. He could not believe the insolence of my questioning. In these moments, his usual recourse was to become philosophical. "That baby in your womb is like a flower budding in the desert, a scorched desert. Now we have to stop the wind, and pray for rain. Do you understand?!" I understood he was calling my womb a desert, and coming from my gynecologist, this was very depressing news indeed.

During one of my routine and increasingly frequent checkups I overheard two doctors speaking in solemn tones about another patient, a pregnant woman who sounded like she was in terrible health. "Previa . . . advanced age . . . advanced endo . . ." How horrible it all sounded! I thought about the poor woman, the complications that would surely come with her rare elderly pregnancy, imagining her brittle bones, her bruised and spotted skin, her body's imminent revolt against itself. Then one of the doctors began to spell the woman's last name, "L-A-K-S-H . . ." *She* was *me*. Those conditions were the titles of *my* miseries. Mine, I learned, was a "geriatric pregnancy."

I knew my pregnancy was high risk. Given my age and the late date at which we finally found out I was really pregnant, I worried about the health of the baby. Had I gotten enough folic acid? Would my endometriosis be a hindrance to the baby's coming out okay? Given the fact that I had only one fallopian tube on one side and one working ovary on the other, had the embryo even implanted properly? So I focused instead on a less dire worry: how to stay active, for my physical and mental health. I've long been a gym rat, and up until that appointment, I had expected to continue my boxing, spinning, and the rest. When Seckin commanded otherwise, I picked his brain for alternatives. Running was a no. So was lifting any weights over a measly three pounds. I couldn't jump or bounce or jostle.

"Can I even walk?" I asked, frustrated.

"Yes, you can walk," he said.

"Well, can I walk up stairs?"

"Yes."

"Aha."

I started on the stairs at the gym, walking up and down the two flights about fifteen to twenty times, but soon stopped. I felt silly and self-conscious, like I was always blocking traffic. Instead, I took to walking the emergency stairs in my apartment building. A fire-exit stairwell, encased in dingy, bare cement walls, connected the floors. There were no windows, no people, no distractions. I walked up slow and steady, skipping one stair with each step. When I traveled for *Top Chef,* Michelle would help me suss out each hotel's emergency stairs.

I listened to music on an iPod at first, but I quickly abandoned music for the rhythmic echo of my footsteps, the cadence of my breath. The stairwell came to serve as a sort of flotation chamber, except that my mind, not my body, needed stilling. Outside of my cement cocoon, my thoughts churned: What am I going to tell people? How am I going to wedge motherhood into my life, then how am I going to wedge my life into motherhood? And how am I going to fit into my clothes?

I admit that I started my slow climbs out of vanity, as a reaction to the desperation I felt when I looked in the mirror and saw my newly bloated body and contourless face. But my daily ascents and descents began to take on a meditative quality. I spent twenty-five to forty-five minutes a day on stairs, depending on the time I had to spare or how much I could bear. Sometimes I realized that the beads of salty water streaking my face were not sweat but tears. It was in these scattered stairwells that I waded through hormone-fueled emotion and egocentric impulse. It was in these stairwells that I came to understand that the time for self-indulgence was over, that my primary purpose now was ensuring the health of the creature growing inside me, that I'd soon be a helpless little person's only succor. I rarely looked forward to a session on the stairs. But once I emerged, blinking at the brightness of the day, I felt happy to have done it.

Then in mid-December, I felt a dull cramping, nothing outrageous or comparable to when I had my period, but definitely there. This startled me because I hadn't had a cramp since becoming pregnant. I called Seckin, who asked me to meet him in his office. When I got there, he determined I was having early contractions and he said we needed to go to the hospital. This rocked me to the core. Up until that time, I had pretty much managed to keep my good humor in spite of everything. But the moment Seckin announced that I might have to be admitted, I felt a sudden helplessness and impotence I had never felt before. An invisible rock formed under my sternum, a heavy ball of dread I could not shake. The ride from Seckin's office to Lenox Hill Hospital is a short one, a mere handful of New York City blocks, but it seemed like an eternity. I felt like a prisoner waiting to be executed.

Adam had yet to decide the correct course of action or determine his desired involvement in the baby's life. On the way to the hospital I phoned to inform him of what was developing. He was in Texas. He did not come to New York.

At the hospital, nurses and other staff struggled to get an IV in me. I became mostly mute and stone-faced as the doctors discussed giving me steroids to expand the baby's lungs in case she did come early. Right now, her lungs weren't developed enough for her to breathe on her own, they explained. They gave me medication to stop the contractions, a drug used for heart patients that worked on the muscles of the heart but also calmed other organs, in my case my uterus. I had extremely low blood pressure, so they monitored not only my heart but the baby's, too. I had pads and patches and tubes taped to various parts of my body and I felt more like a science experiment than a patient. I felt utterly immobilized, paralyzed with fear. I pushed back the only thoughts I had, which were that this was happening because of my emotional callousness. For most of my life I had been a serial monogamist; perhaps this was my punishment for acting like a female Casanova. But why punish the baby? Karma was a big part of my beliefs as a Hindu. So when I first found out about my pregnancy, I immediately attributed it to good karma for starting the foundation with Seckin. Now I considered my current plight also a result of karma. It didn't altogether make sense, and I was afraid of delving even deeper into my thoughts, lest I create some further turmoil in my system. I was too afraid to let my mind wander, and so I mostly stared out the window of my hospital room. People kept bustling in and out for the better part of the rest of that evening.

The drugs eventually calmed my contractions. Seckin and his colleague, another sweet-faced doctor with kind, twinkling eyes named Sam Levin, decided I would get more rest at home. So late into the night I was released. Several days earlier I had given a keynote address at MIT. The Endometriosis Foundation of America had helped to launch a Center for Gynepathology Research there in conjunction with Harvard Medical School. I couldn't believe I was actually standing at a podium in such an institution. We owed much of that success to a biological engineer and professor at MIT named Dr. Linda Griffith, who had read the *Newsweek* interview about my journey with endo and had reached out by cold-calling Seckin's office to see if we could partner on something. She was the real brain and fire behind the center. Dr. Griffith had herself suffered from endometriosis, hiding her illness for years. She even had a couch installed in her office so she could lie down without anyone noticing. She had surgery after surgery, but she told only those closest to her for fear of being passed up for tenure and promotions. She said that reading my story helped her to realize the science and research community needed to devote more resources to the disease. I was just lucky to be standing in the glow of her efforts.

I had also competed in a celebrity charades tournament just days before, and my team had won, beating out other really talented actors and performers. I had been feeling really good, great even. But now I saw that my body could withhold information, that it did not always indicate there was any trouble afoot. It could still dupe and betray me. On Christmas Eve, I began to feel uneasy again. Soon Teddy would be leaving for Africa with his sons and Mukesh Ambani and his family. They were going on safari. Teddy wanted at all costs to improve how his company IMG was functioning around the world, and he needed partners as capable as he was to do so. Mukesh was the person he had handpicked in India. He thought the best way for Mukesh to get to know him better was to go on vacation with him and his family. It was of course too late in my pregnancy for me to fly anywhere, let alone to the heart of Africa. I felt sorry for myself that he was leaving. But my uneasiness took the form of a physical listlessness, a feeling that something was not right. A real growing discomfort. I had trouble getting to sleep and my lower back hurt. There was a general, indescribable ache in my belly, or faint cramping down low. I am not really sure *what* it was that made me feel so out of sorts, so weary and upset. I had been on the phone with Adam a lot, too, in those days, trying to figure things out.

I wound up in the hospital again the day after Christmas with early contractions. This time, I would spend five whole days there. Teddy came to visit me in the hospital before he left. It was the closest I have ever gotten to feeling utterly alone. Manu rode with me in the taxi uptown. As before, I informed Adam. Again, he did not come. My mind was utterly frozen with fear that my child would suffer some defect or handicap due to all the stress I had hoisted upon myself. I felt impotent. I lay there, blinking, with the same belts across my tummy, the fetal heart monitors, the EKG patches, the oxygen and IV tubes.

Sometime after the *New York Post* broke the story that Adam Dell might be the biological father, Adam had decided that he wanted to be fully involved in the baby's life. It felt to me that seeing the news in the paper or online had been some tipping point for him. While prior to that he had said he didn't want to be in the birthing room, now he wanted to be there when the baby was born. I found this ridiculous. I didn't want him in the room. He didn't know about the pregnancy until after the first trimester, but since then he had been absent during almost all of it.

Now, with the distance of time, I can understand the terrible situation Adam found himself in. But back then I really could not. What did the state of affairs between us have to do with his relationship with his child? What happened or didn't happen between the two of us should have nothing to do with his own relationship to the small person-to-be already wiggling around in my belly. Looking back, I can also see that from Adam's view, all he had known firsthand was a traditional family environment. Both his siblings as well as his parents had married young, stayed together for a long time, and produced several kids, in stable, conventional, and happy homes in Texas. He most likely saw his future unfolding in the same way. Now he was forced to see that if he wanted to be a father to his child, this would not be so.

I started to be disappointed in Adam. Each time I informed him I was going to the hospital, I thought for sure that he would come. I had explained to him the danger of the baby coming too early: his own flesh and blood was in peril of not arriving into the world intact and healthy. I was dismayed that he didn't see fit to be there. If not for worry about my safety, at least out of worry for his unborn child. I thought his questions when discussing options sounded selfish. They seemed to be focused on his rights, versus what was best for the baby. At one point he suggested that after the baby was born she and I move to Austin, where I knew no one, had never worked, and would be far away from my friends, family, and Teddy, just to accommodate his personal needs.

I suppose it would have been much easier for all if I had never insisted that Teddy and I conduct that paternity test, but *I* had to know. And I had to make sure our child knew the truth. I didn't want her to grow up not knowing who her father was. It was why, despite everything I still felt, it was vital to have Adam in our child's life as her father. My own personal history and my paternal abandonment compounded the anger I felt at Adam's vacillation.

Krishna was born on a Saturday. It was cold and crisp, and my mother had opened the window in my bedroom to let the cool air in. I had been beached on my bed like a whale for the better part of three months. But even with all the complications and trips to the hospital with fetal heart monitors, et cetera, I felt that I had had a blissful and happy pregnancy. Now I was ready to meet my child, ready to have my body belong primarily to myself again, ready to not sit around like Humpty Dumpty in my bed. Other than my arms, I could only exercise my feet, so I moved them up and down, pointing my toes and then flexing my feet. I did what little I could, but nothing really took away the feeling of being trapped in my own body. I would have jumped out of my skin, except that I was happy for those three months to lie, languorous and perfectly still, a scarab-bodied Cleopatra, because I knew Krishna's life and well-being depended on it. It was easy to do, but enough was enough. I began making little circles in the air with my toes as the early-spring breeze flitted through and puffed the curtains.

There are certain days you know will be strange or special right when you open your blurry eyes. And even though I knew I was to give birth any day very soon, the air felt different, charged. In the morning stillness, when the world is just waking up and your conscious mind hasn't fully taken over, you may feel a connection or passageway to another world, and a feeling that something is about to happen in yours. It's like a quiet storm is coming. You can feel the distant rumble of thunder on the horizon, yet you have no idea of the deluge your life is about to experience. I didn't feel any contractions, but I felt a slow, growing discomfort. Nothing drastic, mind you. But something was there. I was listless, a princess sitting on a pea.

My mother came in with a tray of green tea and honey, grapefruit sprinkled with cinnamon, and an egg in a hole, its round, soft center quivering under a shiny green slick of olive oil. Usually the egg in a hole would be topped with a drizzle of hot sauce or a smattering of pickled jalapeño slices, but with the pregnancy I had experienced heartburn for the first time in my life. So a good coarse cracking of black pepper and sea salt was all I could take. For some reason, I couldn't bring myself to eat today, even though I was hungry. I was playing with my grapefruit when my mother started chastising me. "Eat the egg before it gets cold, *kanna*. And put the tea on your nightstand. It's hot, no? And very full." No matter how close you are to your mother, having her move back in with you at the age of thirty-nine is challenging. We were two women who had been through a lot. Like most mothers and daughters, we had had our share of fights and feasts. The very instincts that made my mother an excellent professional nurse also made her a Herculean mother. She had a knack for taking over completely and relished the role. All of which was mostly fine with me. It was just that sometimes being bossed around when you're a bossy woman yourself is a little frustrating.

I was toying with the gravelly pepper and oil with the side of my knife when I felt a swift kick to my side from deep within. I punctured the yolk and as it oozed its golden richness across the plate I could feel the baby shift. Suddenly I became ravenous and began to sop up the golden fat and white albumen with the crunchy edges of the bread. It was so delicious, I found myself ignoring the baby's kick. Just as I took another perfect bite of egg and toast, olive oil and gritty sea salt, she suddenly decided to shift her body so that I could see my belly literally move under the tray. In a second the tray moved so much that the cup of tea toppled over, sending hot green liquid cascading down the duvet, wetting everything. The cup rolled and bounced off the bed and onto the floor. Damage done, I somehow didn't care. I kept eating that luscious egg.

My mother came in when she heard the teacup hit the wood floor. "Eh! Are you all right, you didn't get burned? I told you to put that cup over there." She rushed in to remove the tray so she could change the wet bedding and rather than thank her, I whined because I wasn't able to sop up the last of the yolky fat on the plate. She asked me to get up and sit in a chair until she cleaned up, and as I did I felt a twinge, a turning inside. But it could have easily been from getting up too fast, or indigestion. I waited and then returned to bed and the twinge came again. I called Seckin, who

egg in a hole

Serves 1

1 to 2 teaspoons extra-virgin olive oil, plus more as needed for the
    pan and for drizzling
1 slice sourdough bread
1 large egg
Fleur de sel
Coarsely ground black pepper

Heat a frying pan over medium heat. Drizzle 1 to 2 teaspoons olive
oil into the pan, distributing it evenly.

Cut a hole about 1 inch in diameter in the center of the bread.
Toast one side of the bread in the pan for 2 to 3 minutes, or until
golden, then flip the bread to the other side, adding a few more drops
of oil if needed. Let the second side toast for another 2 to 3 minutes.

Gently crack the egg into the hole.

Once the egg white is opaque, delicately flip the bread over
with a spatula, being careful not to break the yolk, which should be
nestled in the hole. Cook for a couple more minutes, until the egg is
cooked but the yolk is still quivering slightly. Do not overcook.

Carefully transfer the bread from the pan to a plate and drizzle
with a bit more olive oil. Add a healthy pinch of fleur de sel as well as
4 to 5 turns of a pepper mill over the top. Serve hot.

said I should wait until the contractions got more frequent and severe. He encouraged me to relax, and not to eat too much (too late for that). He suggested I swing a bit in the living room.

A year and a half earlier, I had got it into my head that I wanted a swing in the middle of my living room. Traditional old South Indian homes had swings called *oonjuls* in Tamil or *julas* in Hindi. They were bigger than the American playground swings common in parks. Rectangular planks of rosewood or teak, four to six feet long by almost two feet wide, they were held up by four long, ornately carved brass or iron chains, hooked into rings in the ceiling. Most were used to rock babies to sleep or for reading. A vital part of the Indian wedding ceremony was also performed on these types of swings. Before the tying of the Hindu wedding *thali* and just after exchanging flower garlands, the bridal couple would sit, rocking back and forth in the swing (adorned especially with flowers, too, for the occasion), signifying the waves of life the couple would experience together in harmony. All the women on both sides of the couple form a semicircle around the pair. They sing love songs, specific Sanskrit songs that everyone knows, blessing the couple to have a long, happy married life. Usually the women with the best voices get pushed to the front. In places of honor, the mothers-in-law or women really close to the couple slowly wave a plate of flowers, rice with turmeric and vermillion powder, as well as a ritualistic flame round and round in front of the couple.

Rajima's Tanjore home, nestled between coconut groves and the banks of the Kaveri River, had at least one such swing. I remember sitting on it as she dried my wet hair by smoking it over a small pot of hot coals sprinkled with a fragrant resin called *sambrani,* made from the dried bark of styrax trees, after we bathed in the river with tiny fish nibbling at our toes. *Sambrani* is often burned to calm the nerves and induce tranquility, especially in children, and to prepare the atmosphere for prayer or any auspicious occasion by purifying the air.

I didn't have any *sambrani*. But I did have a swing. Adam had built me a little wooden one back in 2008, connecting blue velvet-covered ropes into iron rings in my wood-beamed ceiling. So in order to calm myself, and the contractions, I swung. My mother disappeared into the pantry to say a prayer and light some incense at the *puja* altar. I swung, higher and higher in all my roundness. I looked down at the little round shape jutting out from my oblong oval belly, clearly the baby's butt sticking out to the side. Soon she would be out. Soon there would be two of us. Regardless of what happened, I wanted to savor these final blissful moments. I thought of KCK telling me, "You are American now, you must live like they live," but inside I still felt very Indian. I sang old Carnatic songs off-key and often with patches of jumbled sounds when I couldn't remember the right lyrics. This baby would most likely be very American. I could not say how much of my own heritage, diluted by time and geography, would trickle down to her. Would she have my mother's deep Cupid's bow upper lip, like I did? Would she have the big, rounded forehead my grandfather passed down to us all?

Maryanne, my beloved friend and acupuncturist, came by to administer a treatment as we had planned and found me on the swing. She could not have been more pleased. She needled me on my green couch, the same one I had sat in when the fertility specialist told me my ovaries were older than I was, and then promptly sent me back to the swing. I was still swinging when Teddy arrived at my door. "There's your favorite apple crumble pie warming in the oven," I said. I didn't want it to spoil if I got stuck in the hospital, so I'd decided to heat it up while I was swinging. There were enough of us around, so I ordered pizza from my favorite joint on Avenue B, too. "Junior, you are original in all you do. *Sui generis!* Jeez, how can you think of food right now? And will you get off that swing, you're making me queasy."

I went to the hospital that afternoon with my mother and Maryanne in the backseat, driven by Dr. Seckin himself. Teddy followed in his car. I was pretty calm. I knew I wanted my mother there as well as Maryanne, so she could administer acupuncture for pain control (I wanted to be awake for the birth even if it was an emergency C-section) as well as to harvest my placenta and carry it out of the hospital safely. I wanted Teddy in the room for various reasons. One, I felt the most calm and safe when Teddy was around. And two, although he was squeamish, I knew he would be a wonderful partner. Teddy was always a great clutch player. That's who you want near you when times get tough. Teddy had the heart of a firefighter. When others rushed away, he rushed in to save the day. I also wanted him to experience the birth hand in hand with me. He certainly deserved it. I felt it was one of the few things he had never had the chance to experience in his long and colorful life. I was more than happy to give him that experience. He didn't disappoint. He was a rock. He was funny. He made me focus and be thankful that this moment had indeed come. The mere fact that he was still by my side gave me great strength.

My cousin Manu phoned Adam just about the time I went into labor, when Seckin decided it was not a fire drill but the real thing. The baby was coming. By coincidence, my cousin Vinod and his partner, Tim, were driving down from Albany for the weekend, so they were in town. I also had extra aunts in from India, who added to the number of relatives who would eventually show up at Lenox Hill. Later that day, at 5:59 p.m., Krishna was born. I remained awake for as long as it took to remove her from my belly. Dr. Seckin held her up. I remember thinking she looked like a long stalk of buttered white asparagus. He gave her to Teddy, who brought her to me.

Those first few hours were a groggy blur. The only thing I remember clearly is the moment Teddy brought Krishna to me. I thought my heart would burst with happiness. I remember staring into his face as he held my hand. In the moment just before we heard her cry, I looked up at him and said I was scared. "Of what, Junior? There's nothing to be frightened of." I said I didn't know and he replied, "Just remember our life is about her now." What struck me at that moment was how this man could love me so resolutely, after everything. How he had said "our" and not "your" life. I burst into tears and laughter as I heard Krishna's first cry. It sounded small, almost like a kitten mewling, nothing like those boisterous cries you hear from newborns in movies. Teddy took the baby out to my mother, who had been patiently waiting along with almost every other member of my family. Nine eager brown faces waited, all squished in the tiny waiting area for this long-bodied little pale face with squinty eyes and rosy cheeks.

I had purposely checked into the hospital under an assumed name. But the next day my publicist called me to let me know that she had received several inquiries from various press outlets and so she commented that the baby, named Krishna Thea, and I were both fine, as I had instructed her in advance to do if she was asked by more than three separate outlets. Apparently the news got out that I had given birth because Seckin had arrived late to a neighbor's dinner party and apologized to the host, letting her know why. He thought he was having a private conversation, but an editor from *Food & Wine* magazine, also present, overheard and tweeted this sensitive information to the world. Poor old Seckin was mortified when I spoke with him about it afterward.

Adam flew in from Texas the day after Krishna was born. He saw and held the baby for the first time at Lenox Hill. He kept saying how "light" she was. At first I thought he meant her weight, but he meant the color of her skin. We were all expecting a brown-eyed, tawny-skinned little thing with jet-black Asian hair to appear and instead, out came this pale white baby with blue eyes and downy light-brown hair. Adam kept calling me the morning of the third day, agitating to come to the hospital again. I mistook it for enthusiasm, not anger. The night before, we had had a good visit. I even nursed the baby while he and his father remained in the room without asking them to leave. I asked him to come after Seckin examined me, which was to be in the late morning, so he could have an uninterrupted visit. He kept calling to see if the doctor had been in. And I repeatedly said he hadn't yet. Then Seckin finally did arrive, and he asked me to lift my gown and spread my legs so he could examine my stitches. The doctor had just put his gloves on and began to examine me when the door to my hospital room flung open without a knock. Adam and his dad started to walk in when Seckin, startled, raised his arm and asked them to wait outside. Seckin looked me in the eye for a really long time as if to say, "Are you all right?" Once my exam had finished, Adam and his dad entered again. Adam towered over my bed. His face was colored deep pink, and his ears seemed to be getting red. He asked me why I didn't include his name in the announcement, and at first I had zero idea of what he was talking about. I was still quite out of it, feeling the effects of anesthesia and post-op sedation. I was exhausted from the birth. But I remember crying, and asking Adam not to yell at me. He exited the room several times, running to the nurses' station, demanding to see the birth certificate. They told him the registrar, not anyone in the maternity ward, had it. He went down to the registrar's office but they said they had sent it in to the county.

The papers, it turned out, had printed Krishna's name as Krishna Thea Lakshmi. This enraged Adam. I did not know why this became such an alarming thing for him at that very moment. If indeed he became involved in Krishna's life, we could always add his name. My birth certificate has my birth father's surname, but no one even knew or cared. I took my mom's last name, Lakshmi, because she was my primary caregiver. It seemed that Adam was focusing on marking territory, on symbolism with no substance.

He could not control his temper. In spite of his father and my mother trying to calm him down he could not lower his voice or speak normally to me. And this while the baby was in the room. In Indian culture, we believe that whatever you expose the child to in the first few weeks and months of life will have a profound effect on her. I was concerned that the baby would absorb the negative energy coming from Adam. The atmosphere was horrible.

He kept pacing ominously back and forth in my tiny room, refusing to sit down. After a few hours of this, his father finally convinced him to leave and escorted him out. I was shaken to the core. I couldn't believe that someone, let alone my baby's very father, could behave that way mere hours after I had given birth. I had thought he would know that behaving in such a way was foolish and arrogant and totally inappropriate. Didn't he know that this moment, this tender beginning for all of us, would now be sullied by his bullying?

We hadn't even come to any final decisions on anything. Furthermore, why shouldn't my last name be fine to give the baby? Millions of people around the world bear their father's last name, and it didn't mean that they loved their mother any less. So why was it so offensive that she just have mine? Was mine alone not good enough? This raised my feminist ire as well as my ancestral matriarchal streak. What did it matter what the papers said anyway? It all seemed to be, yet again, a focus on nothing of importance or depth at that moment. I hadn't even publicly acknowledged who the father was, and had no plans to release such personal information, given that we had not reached any agreement. For the rest of my stay at Lenox Hill, I had hospital security escort my mom with the baby in her plexiglas gurney to another, empty hospital room so Krishna could visit with her father.

I was very worried I wouldn't be able to nurse Krishna. After Adam's blowup in the hospital, I spoke very few words to him. I wanted him nowhere near me. In those first days of Krishna's life, my milk began to dry up after coming in fine for the first few feedings. I worried that the stress of the altercation in the hospital had caused it to diminish. Thankfully, it returned, but not ever to the level of those mothers who are lucky enough to be able to freeze or express it in advance.

chapter 14

The decision to consume my own placenta was not an easy one.
Sometime during my pregnancy Maryanne brought the issue
up when I said how terrified I was of going back to work six weeks after
giving birth. The schedule of filming *Top Chef* is quite grueling by any standards, but the nice part is that after working pretty much round the clock
for a month and a half, I am pretty free except for filming the finale, which
comes months later.

Still, days on the show, especially in the first half of a season, can last
fifteen or sixteen hours. I had been bedridden for six weeks before the baby
came and was told to stay in bed six weeks after to heal. I was now up at all
hours and nursing as well. I was worried I would collapse from exhaustion
once filming began. Combined with the long hours were the marathons
of eating on the set. My digestive tract would take a beating and debilitate
my energy further. Maryanne brought up the fact that many mothers ate
the nutritious tissue of their placenta as a way to shore up their energy
reserves. Eating the placenta fortified her clients' health and stamina and
generally aided in their getting up and running normally much faster. The
primary benefit, however, was warding off postpartum depression, some-

thing I feared more than fatigue. And I had had bouts of depression myself at various times in my life.

Maryanne had already filled out a lot of paperwork with the hospital ahead of time so she could minister to me in my room during the time of or just before my delivery. I wanted acupuncture for pain control as well as to calm my stress levels. We didn't know how the delivery would go and I was adamant about staying awake for Krishna's coming. So Maryanne had permission to be there. Once the baby came out safely, a nurse in the OR collected the expelled placenta, placed it in a white plastic container commonly used for organ transplants, and handed Maryanne my biological waste. Maryanne placed the container in a brown shopping bag, calmly walked directly out of the hospital, and caught a cab downtown to my showroom and test kitchen in Alphabet City.

There, she placed the placenta in the fridge and went to Kmart with my assistant, Tucker. They bought all new knives, cutting boards, baking sheets, a coffee grinder, a pot for boiling, and a strainer, as well as disposable gloves. The next day, after a lengthy process that led to powdered placenta, Maryanne and Tucker used a tiny funnel and many little gelatin capsules to parcel out small daily doses of my very life force. I left strict instructions for them to throw out every single utensil and pan afterward. I told no one outside of those involved what had taken place in our studio or what the content of my little pills was until many months later.

I didn't really feel comfortable at the time about the project, but I would have done anything to defend myself against collapsing from stress and fatigue or succumbing to the postpartum depression I was so afraid would beset me. Given the ever-present white noise of the drama and tension surrounding visitation rights and questions of custody happening between me and Adam, as well as the media scrutiny into very private matters in my life, depression was a constant threat. So resorting to encapsulated cannibalism did not seem so sinister to me.

Now, a couple of years on, I'm quite proud of eating my placenta. Our own bodies can give us a lot. I felt self-reliant and earthy, but of course I had not been the one standing there at the stove watching my flesh boil. I was thankful I had trusted friends and colleagues who would do it for me. Later, many months after the pills ran out, I did suffer from severe depression and asked my doctors for all the peer-reviewed articles pertaining to research on taking antidepressants while breast-feeding. Since I did not find much, I chose to refrain from taking any. I would breast-feed for a year and eight months. Most of that time, it would be a struggle to collect enough milk to sustain Krishna. Another plan of attack was hatched for that. Pills and tinctures, of milk thistle, blessed thistle, fenugreek or fennel seed, and garlic boiled in milk; constant massage; and drinking three to four liters of water a day all played a part in coaxing my body to do its job.

The finale of the DC season filmed in Singapore when Krishna was almost six months old. That July, we packed up to go to Asia. I had never fed Krishna anything but my own milk or the occasional top-up with formula when I had problems making enough to satisfy her growing hunger. The lucky coincidence of being that close to India during this time meant that Krishna would be able to have her first food ceremony, or *annaprasanam*, in Chennai at Rajima's house. When I had informed Neela that I thought Krishna would soon be ready to eat something solid (she had been drooling at me with big eyes every time I lifted spoon to mouth lately) and asked what I should give her first, she stopped me cold. "Vait, vait, *vait!!* You can't just give her food on your own! Jima will kill you, this close to India especially?! You have to bring her here, we have to call the priests, and *then* you can give her some small bit of rice and *dal*, or *kichidi*, but no black pepper, of course, just some *jeera*." What about my grandpa's famous banana *payasam*? I was looking forward to Krishna tasting that.

Pongal, or *kichidi*, as it's called in the north, is a simple white rice and mung lentil porridge that is made with very little else but butter and cumin

kichidi

Serves 4 to 6

1 cup yellow or orange (masoor)* lentils

½ cup white basmati rice

2 fresh bay leaves

1 teaspoon salt, plus ½ teaspoon more for seasoning the vegetables

2 tablespoons canola oil

¼ teaspoon cumin seeds

½ cup chopped shallots

2 tablespoons minced fresh ginger

½ cup diced red bell pepper

½ cup diced carrots

½ teaspoon Madras or sambar curry powder

1 cup chopped fresh baby spinach leaves

½ cup chopped fresh cilantro

1 tablespoon butter

½ teaspoon coarsely crushed black peppercorns

8 to 10 fresh curry leaves

* *Moong lentils are also fine, as they are usually used in traditional versions of kichidi.*

Rinse the lentils and rice until the water runs clear, and transfer them to a big stockpot. Add the bay leaves and salt and cover with 2 to 3 inches of water and stir. Bring to a boil, reduce heat to medium, and cook for 25 to 30 minutes, skimming off any foam that appears during cooking. Stir occasionally to prevent sticking. Add a bit more water, if needed.

Meanwhile, heat the oil in a skillet over medium heat. Add the cumin seeds. After a minute, when the cumin starts to sizzle, add the shallots and ginger. Stir. When the shallots become glassy, after about 4 to 5 minutes, add the bell pepper and the carrots and stir to sauté. Add ½ teaspoon salt and the curry powder. Stir, cooking for 3 to 5 minutes more, until the vegetables are done but still al dente. Remove from heat and cover to keep warm. Once the lentil-and-rice mixture is ready, add the sautéed vegetables. Stir together. Remove from heat.

Now add the spinach and cilantro, stirring well. Adjust salt to taste. In a separate pan, melt the butter. Add the black peppercorns and cook over low heat just until fragrant and slightly browned. Once the butter is golden brown, add the curry leaves. Fry for 30 seconds or less.

Drizzle the butter mixture on top of the *kichidi* and serve warm. It should have a porridge-like consistency.

—•••—

or a few peppercorns and peas. It may have a scant few other cut vegetables in it, but it is mostly supposed to be purposefully bland and comforting for when you are ill or have stomach problems. It can be served with plain yogurt on the side and perhaps some spicy condiment or pickle, but for the most part is a neutral and wholesome dish eaten by Indians all over the world. Our version of chicken soup, perhaps. In the last trimester of my pregnancy, when I became grounded and often suffered from extreme acidity, I began to eat copious amounts of the stuff. In my modernized version of the recipe, I inverted the proportions of rice to lentils, two cups of lentils for every cup of rice, instead of the other way around. I wanted to have the traditional Indian comfort food, but with more protein and less starch. I also substituted more flavorful orange *masoor* lentils for the pale yellow *moong.* I added a heap of various vegetables, from shredded lacinato kale, chopped celery, and fennel bulb to julienned carrots and finely chopped cauliflower. I added freshly minced ginger and sautéed it with some diced shallots, too. This recipe, the most comforting one I know, also helped me lose the baby weight. I lived on bowls and bowls of it while nursing.

But I knew that this recipe was not my grandmother's *pongal.* I knew I could not suggest anything other than what they prescribed for Krishna's special day. "Oh, of course, it's very important what her first food is," I said, feigning innocence. A deep, long silence on the phone from Neela seemed to be screaming: *ARE YOU CRAZY?* "Just get here and we will handle the rest."

While we did observe most major holidays, our family in India was for the most part pretty secular. So I didn't know what the sudden fire drill was about. I had really no recollection of what *annaprasanam* was, to be frank. Simply put, it is the ritual to commemorate the baby's budding relationship to food, to bless a child with lifelong good dietary habits and much bounty in her life. It marks the transition from mother's milk to real food; from liquid to solids. This was my kind of ceremony. How could I have missed it? Who doesn't like a celebration of food? Well, I was young when it happened to me, and just eight when it happened to Rohit, the last of the births in our generation that I was there for. So I could be forgiven for not remembering.

But I did know enough to sense that what had recently happened at a Singaporean strip mall while we were shooting was not, well . . . kosher. Every location we shot *Top Chef* in had some "must-try" down-and-dirty local joint for tacos or dumplings or barbeque. Wherever the place, all of us made a mental list of the things we needed to try and often passed that info around the set through word of mouth and call sheets, memos, and texts. Part of the fun of a traveling food show is getting to try all these interesting, off-the-wall edibles in situ. Singapore was a cornucopia of pan-Asian food, from fresh live frogs fried to order with salt and white pepper sauce at the No Signboard restaurant, to hawkers who sold sizzling satay off their street carts at nighttime. Our crew took pleasure in sampling it all. I was no different, and prided myself on being quite a culinary spelunker.

Traveling to distant lands and consuming whatever local delicacies they offered was my preferred way of life. My modeling career, and even before that, crisscrossing the world to go between my mom's home in the U.S. and my grandmother's home in India, had afforded me many opportunities along the way to sample the food in other countries. In fact, I had been to Singapore alone several times on my way to Madras before the age of eighteen. So when the camera guys told us about the dumpling house in the food court just half a mile from our hotel, my assistant, Jason, Michelle, and I *had* to go. One afternoon after a Quickfire shoot had finished, I nursed the baby and attached her to my chest in the Baby Bjorn. And off we went to the mall. We ordered exactly what we were told was the specialty: various dumplings in a beef broth soup. The restaurant was more fast-food dive in the middle of a bustling food court at the tail end of the lunch hour than proper establishment, and looked like an old repurposed Panda Express, with neon lighting and plastic laminated white and light-blue Formica tables. I grew up reading Calvin Trillin and all his food adventures. I was also used to eating in all kinds of places, so this did not faze me in the least and I brought Krishna along. We waited patiently, Krishna dangling from my torso, cooing and jiving to the crowds of people and sights around her.

Once the bowls of steaming soup came, I gently ladled a sip onto a big ceramic Chinese spoon, careful to graze off any hot, scalding drops of broth that may have been hanging from the bottom to protect Krishna's head. I held the spoon absentmindedly in front of me—but of course in front of the baby, too. As I listened to whatever joke Jason was making, waiting for my broth to cool, Krishna leaned in and began to slurp what was on the spoon. I could see her head crane and turn sideways as I guided the spoon up and over her head toward my waiting mouth for every subsequent bite. We all thought this was funny. "No, no, no, this isn't for you! You haven't even had cow's milk yet, never mind cow meat or broth!" We Hindus believe that the first thing you feed a child is incredibly important. Traditionally, Brahmin Hindus do not eat any meat or eggs. I never thought this would be how Krishna would eat, growing up in the West. But I suddenly felt a pang of guilt. *You are giving her the soup from the carcass of a cow, our most sacred animal.* There were so many customs and observances of my upbringing that I had been unable to fulfill, but this one, however, I was totally aware of from a very early age. I had a plan in mind for Krishna's diet, a precise one. Vegetables and grains slowly introduced one by one, in succession, after she turned six months old. No animal products whatsoever until after age one, and then only dairy, and then eggs, but only after eighteen months. Then fish and seafood after age two, and chicken at two and a half, then red meat after that but only if she took a liking to it.

Murky beef broth with floating bits of mystery meat was not what I had in mind as her first foray into real food! I felt horrible that literally under my nose, in that moment, I had undone the best-laid plans of a cornerstone of my duties as her mother. Not to mention that I had effectively denied my heritage and disregarded the practices of my own religion. I prided myself on how well one could eat following a Hindu Brahmin lacto-vegetarian diet. I had extolled its virtues on many occasions and truly believed in its merits. I knew that what had happened, while an accident, was also karmic retribution for all the bodies of animals I had consumed in my life and career in food. I felt a horrible knot in my stomach that was half guilt and half dread, bound together with a glue of feeling like a fool for not understanding that of course Krishna would be tempted. Whose daughter was she, anyway?

Michelle tried to put a positive spin on the first-food fiasco. "Well, at least she is willing to try new things!" "Just pretend it didn't happen," Jason countered. "You can't blame a little baby, and you only looked away for a second." I knew I would roast in some far-off Hindu hell for not adhering to the easiest of rules of my faith's culinary tenets. But then, shortly after, curiosity overtook guilt and any sense of duty. I wanted to see if it was a fluke or not, so I did the unthinkable, the blasphemous. I gave her a second spoonful. "Okay, now you're asking for it; I am looking the other way because I don't want to lie to your mom when she asks me if you ever fed KT anything you shouldn't have," Michelle said. She was scared of my mom and had had the pleasure of her unwavering company for the entirety of our DC filming. After the third spoonful, I quit out of fear that it would upset the baby's tummy. I was sure that diarrhea or colic would be the poetic retribution for my flouting the precepts of proper Hindu dietary habits. It would serve me right, I thought. Poor little Krishna, she had to sit there and watch us slurp the famous dumplings I cannot even remember the taste of now.

All the women in my family were psychotically particular about when and what foods you fed babies and children at every stage of their development. And I was about to get an earful from my grandma about the dos and don'ts of how to feed the newest member of our family. "Start with something savory, *not* sweet, as is often the custom, even among some of the extended members of our family," Rajima sniffed. My grandmother felt that whatever food you first gave the baby would imprint itself upon her palette and establish certain expectations and tastes throughout her existence. Teach a child the pleasures of eating well, and you affect that child for the rest of her life. Feed her sugar first, and the danger is that she will always come to expect it with every meal. For a race more prone to diabetes than any other, this was a perilous situation. And also, "Don't go giving the baby everything in your big American fridge," they admonished. Introduce one food at a time, cooked at home with just a pinch of salt. No tomatoes. No citrus. And whatever you do, *do not give this child store-bought baby food.*

The advent of bottled and packaged baby food is, in my opinion, why many children have a hard time eating well when they graduate to real food in the United States. Most store-bought baby food has no mouth appeal, and certainly no flavor to speak of. While there are some nice new brands out there that strive to address the concerns of parents who want everything organic and cruelty-free and locally sourced, the actual appeal and taste of the food in question remains dismal. Somewhere along the line, after World War II, we were brainwashed into believing that we needed some multinational corporation to give us the food that was most wholesome and good for our progeny. We were conditioned to think that the big food brands knew better than we did what was best for our little ones, and that the food coming out of factories was superior to the food coming out of our own kitchens. Also, with more and more mothers entering the workforce during the 1970s and 1980s, it became that much easier for us to hand jars rather than recipes to those who cared for our children while we were away at work.

But convenience aside, it's much less expensive for us to make our own food. I remember being on Andy Cohen's show with a former actress who had made a newly minted career for herself by extolling her philosophies on raising children in a kind manner. She once talked publicly (and regretted it later) of chewing up her baby's food in her own mouth and feeding it to her child. While that seems extreme (I wondered why she didn't just invest in an immersion or hand blender), I couldn't help but think that as a society we have gotten so far from what is natural that a person who espoused regurgitating food was actually seen as sane and a viable way for the pendulum to swing back.

It is so easy to give your children good nutrition as well as an appreciation of what good food is just by exposing them to it at an earlier age. The dirty truth is that many adult Americans don't eat right and actually know it. That bottle of puce-colored strained peaches and pumpkin (one we'd never eat ourselves) gets handed to the unsuspecting baby out of fear and convenience. And before you know it, that child out in the real world discovers fried chicken nuggets with ketchup or pizza and doesn't want to eat anything else. Who can blame her?

All of this sanctimonious pontificating does not at all, by the way, excuse or explain why I gave Krishna beef broth that day. Later, on that sunny summer day in Chennai, it also added deep stress and a guilty docility to the proceedings of her *annaprasanam* ceremony. "You must control what food your child eats, and make sure only you or someone you trust touches that food. And don't make the mistake of giving your baby bland food." "Increase the seasonings slowly and gently, adding things like cumin and ginger when appropriate, or your child will forever be one of those boring people who doesn't like anything but the most pedestrian of dishes." "A person's palate is like anything else, it must be trained, stimulated, cultivated, and buffered." I certainly got an earful.

"So if we aren't giving *payasam* or *kheer*, what should we make for the *puja*?" I asked. I was really craving my Tha-Tha's *payasam*; the smell of camphor and incense ignited a Pavlovian rumble in my tummy for the pleasing taste of starchy-sticky soft banana lumps, mashed into cardamom-infused, sweet, cold milk. "*Pongal. Kichidi,*" Rajima pronounced. "That's what she will have." "I told you," Neela mouthed behind her. "No sugar in the first bite. We can give her a small square of *kalkund* or rock candy at the end maybe; we will need that, too, anyway, for the *puja*, but only at the end."

Suddenly, I didn't feel like a grown woman with a child, but a child who had to be guided every step of the way through a dark culinary forest, lest I make some irrevocable mistake. I was told exactly what we were going to do, and I had no choice in the matter. I was informed by Rajima and Bhanu that *they* would pressure-cook the rice and lentils separately, and then *they* would be mashing the two together by hand with a little salt, and a mere few cumin seeds, *not* peppercorns, of course. Of course!

I usually went along with whatever these women told me to do over the years, sometimes out of laziness, other times out of diplomacy. But this was my baby, and I wanted to have a hand in everything that happened to her. Why were they marginalizing me? Did they somehow know of our little transgression at the Singapore mall? Plus, I think I know a thing or two about food, after all. Still, in that house, on that green tile, I instantly became a child again, waiting for instructions on how not to break my new doll.

It was decided after speaking to our priests that the ceremony would be done the following Saturday morning. First, the floor would be swept and washed well before sunrise. Then Neela would draw a traditional *kollam* or *rangoli*, a floral and geometric design made with flour and water paint, on the floor and let it dry. On top of that, a six-inch-high square pit would be made by stacking bricks to house the sacred fire in front of which the priests would recite Sanskrit Vedic prayers. My uncle Vichu, dressed in his Brahmin best of white *veshti* cloth and homespun kurta, would bring the fruits: whole small bananas and brown bearded coconuts set on silver plates before the ceremonial fire, along with little bowls my aunt Bhanu filled with vermillion powder, sandalwood paste, and *vibhuti* ash for our foreheads, and raw rice and little squares of rock candy that looked like a glittering brunoise of quartz crystal. There were flowers in platters and rosewater in a silver tumbler with an ornate spoon to pour it into the fire at the precise moment you were instructed to do so. A small brigade of priests, clothed in nothing but draped and twisted gold-edged white cotton and a sacred Brahmin thread draped across bare chests, with their foreheads smeared with three horizontal lines of *vibhuti*, would file into our home shortly after 9:00 a.m.

The only task I was relegated to perform was to get myself and Krishna bathed and dressed on time. I was instructed to give her the first early-morning feeding but skip the 9:00 a.m. one so that she would be sufficiently hungry to open her mouth at the right moment in the ceremony. I never knew the baby to lack an appetite, but I knew when Jima meant business and so I didn't dare veer off plan for a second.

Neela had laid out a beautiful Madras plaid multicolored silk sari and blouse on the bed for me and even picked out Krishna's outfit. It had taken me longer than usual to bathe Krishna that morning. Our bathroom consisted of two taps for hot and cold that filled up tall plastic buckets waiting below them. You had to wash standing up, using a mug to splash water on you, stop and soap yourself, and then rinse the same way. You could always hear when the neighbors were bathing next door because of the hard splash a mug of water made on the South Indian tile. I tried to keep Krishna contained by immersing her in one of the buckets. It was as tall as she was. This bought me a bit of time to shampoo my own hair without worrying about stinging her eyes while she splashed in her bucket. I had to quickly get both of us clean without monopolizing the hot water intended to serve the whole family. You could never perform a *puja* or any religious ceremony without freshly washing your hair and bathing. In fact, you weren't even allowed to go to the temple when you had your period, as you were considered unclean. I always wondered how anyone would know, quite frankly. But then I guess God would know; as he or she surely knew about the beef broth!

We oiled Krishna's body, and she squealed and squirmed like a wet seal. She had silver-belled anklets in those days, so you always knew when she was awake or moving. She kicked into the air like she knew there was some excitement that centered solely on her. The ease of her age meant that I could place her in the center of the bed and while she could turn herself over, she was unable to move too much and therefore was safe. My brightly colored sari in intersecting squares of orange, midnight-blue, green, and mustard-yellow rustled around me as I used too many pins to secure it for an Indian woman my age. My grandmother and the aunts in my family wouldn't stoop to using any pins, but on this day I wanted to make sure my sari did not unravel in front of the priests. I quickly made the accordion folds in the center of my waist and tucked the pleats into my petticoat. I tied my hair back with fresh garlands of fragrant jasmine and put a small black adhesive *bindi* on Krishna's forehead. She looked adorable, an amalgam of East and West, with sparkling light eyes and fair Caucasian skin molded onto recognizably Indian features and robed in gold brocade with burgundy-and-mustard-colored silk with her anklets jingling. When I had taken her to the temple the night before, full on a Friday evening, people pointed and called her "Gerber baby," like the child in those baby-food ads with downy light hair and a cherubic smile. I found this funny and mortifying all at once.

Outside our bedroom, which used to belong to Rajni and her parents, I could hear the hustle and bustle of preparations. I could hear my uncle Vichu's voice asking my grandma if there was anything to munch on. "You'll eat after the baby eats," she scolded. A stroke she suffered several years ago had thwarted the dexterity in her right hand and arm, but had not diminished anything else to date. She was still ruling our roost with absolute authority. I was getting hungry, too. I could smell the *puja* fire and camphor being ignited. I could hear the jingle of a priest's brass bell and his booming voice as he cleared his throat and gave orders about the proper placement of vessels to a younger priest.

Soon I heard chanting and the familiar call of Rajima: "Padma, eh Padma! *Inga va, velleela va!*" "Come out here now," she beckoned, not much different from when I was late for the St. Michael's school bus. I smeared some kohl into my eyes and ran out with the baby. Outside in the living room sat the members of my family, of this old household, who were left in

Chennai. In front of them were three priests in semicircle formation around the fire, on the embellished floor. I was instructed to sit at my uncle's feet, with Neela on one side and Bhanu on the other. Krishna was placed on my lap and made to lie across. All of us were in our formal Benares silk saris and the heat and smoke from the *puja* fire were getting to me, making my eyes sting and water. With the chanting, the smell of incense, the fire and commotion, and being engulfed in the middle of a dazzling tangle of all our colorful saris, Krishna became fussy. She began to uncharacteristically wriggle and cry. While it worried me, it did not so much as ruffle Rajima. When I looked up at her, she immediately sensed what I was thinking. She raised her hand, bony fingers spread. "Don't worry. She is supposed to cry. Her life will never be the same. You can't give her everything."

I realized what Rajima meant. Until that moment, I had been almost exclusively providing everything Krishna could want or need. I was her sole succor and haven. But her needs were changing. She would now need sustenance from the earth, from Mother Nature, from the world, or at least Whole Foods. She would need more than what I could give her from my own body. We prayed for Krishna to have a bountiful world around her always, for her to have health, and abundance, for her to have plenty. We prayed for her to have a good, wholesome relationship with what feeds her.

But in that moment, I prayed for her to always need me. I prayed to whatever god we were all chanting to, to always be able to feed her, if not from my breast then from the fruits of my own labor. I prayed for a full hand whenever I raised it to Krishna's mouth. I was acutely aware of all the people in this room and across oceans who had helped me through the most difficult transition of my life. I had not taken the path to motherhood alone. Outside, I heard the crows caw in the big tabebuia tree that shaded the veranda. For a second I imagined I even heard the echo of my grandfather singing hymns in his old creaky wicker chair, but I knew that couldn't be so. It was probably someone else's grandpa down the lane. The sun came in through the open veranda door. The heat was rising fast. It was almost 10:00 a.m.

My grandmother emerged with a small *katori*, or bowl, with mashed-up lentils and rice from the kitchen. Her hand, wrinkled and worn, had mixed rice for every child of our family in this house for over thirty-five years. It was the same hand that had braided and oiled my hair, drawn countless marks of vermillion on my forehead, and had even landed hard on the side of my thigh when needed. This hand had shown Neela how to pleat her sari, and Bhanu the right way to burp Rajni and Rohit. It was the same hand that mixed batches of our secret house recipe for *sambar* curry powder twice a year, wielded the ladle of *dosa* batter when I first learned to make the fluffy thin crepes on the iron griddle, and administered Tiger Balm to KCK's temples in the days when his head ached from the monsoon heat.

For a moment, I thought she might be the one to feed Krishna herself. I was keeping a low profile, doing as I was told. After handing me the bowl, she bent over, with agility, impossibly low, and applied a line of holy *vibhuti* ash across Krishna's forehead as she lay writhing in annoyance. "*Ippo, nee punnu,*" Rajima said. "Now you do it." Then I heard my mother's voice, coming from a table where an open laptop was perched. She was tuning in via Skype and commanding me from Los Angeles. "Come on, Pads, the baby's hungry!" I snapped to attention and placed a small espresso spoon of *kichidi* into the baby's mouth. At first she coughed and sputtered but in mere seconds, she seemed to be mashing the pap with her tongue against the roof of her mouth like an old toothless man. Everyone in the room seemed to exhale at once. I heard the hearty belly laughs of the priests.

I thought then that for the first time in my life, in that house, these women were finally saying: "Okay, you're up. It's your turn." For the first time, I did not feel like a minor, a junior, or a half pint. For the women in my family, I had finally made it to full adulthood, into their club, the big league. For a second I mourned not only the final extinguishing of my girlhood, but the further separation, though ever so slight, between my body and Krishna's.

The two things I remember about every important day or evening of my life are what I wore and what I ate. In fact, I can say with great conviction that food has played a central role not only in my professional but also in my emotional life, in all of my dealings with loved ones and most of all in my relationship to myself and my body. I am what feeds me. And how I feed myself at any given moment says a lot about what I'm going through or what I need. I don't believe I am alone. Yes, we eat for our stomachs, but we hunger with our hearts. Like most people and many women, I think about what to eat all the time. I am constantly plotting my next meal, planning how and what I will shop for, and ever hatching new plans to avoid the foods I know will undermine my well-being. Foods are like men: some are good, some are bad, and some are okay only in small doses. But most should be tried at least once.

Since I can remember, people have asked me the same question: How do I eat so much and stay slim? The answer is simple: a lot of hard work. Much of the work is physical, some of it mental, all of it involving vast amounts of willpower and discipline I don't always have. A good chunk is emotional and intuitive. One of the biggest moments in my life in food was a quiet one. An internal event, silent and profound, it happened about a month after childbirth, when I hadn't lost any of the forty-five pounds I had gained. I had expected to bounce back, with moderate exercise and breast-feeding. But I hadn't bounced back at all. In fact, I had gained six and a half pounds—the weight of my new baby—in the two weeks *after* giving birth. In that moment, I understood that the most important part of "getting my body back" was not going to be exercising, or the discipline to do it after I had been up all night and worked all day. It was not going to be portion control or exerting the willpower it took not to reach for cookies or pizza. It was not even the time it would take to prepare healthy meals or count calories. Although I did do all of that, as much as I humanly could.

It was going to have to be the emotional work that got not only my body back, but also my confidence. I just decided that I wasn't going to be upset if I didn't lose the weight. I didn't expect miracles and I was fine with being my new size. My baby was the miracle. My body had given me the greatest gift, one that I had been told I shouldn't hope for. I was not going to feel bad about how I looked or expect to fulfill some vain image I had of myself. After a lifetime of being in front of the camera, I had to give up relying on my figure as a source of status, even if making my living still involved my physical appearance somewhat. So I became consciously pragmatic about the expectations I put on my body, on my self. I was truly, deeply okay with not losing the weight, in case that was what turned out to be my future.

It took a great amount of soul-searching and humility to come to terms with the fact that the good old days were gone and might not return again. That's not to say I didn't hope that all the other things I was doing would pay off. But I wasn't like other models and colleagues who walked the runway in their skivvies eight days after giving birth. I didn't appear on the cover of a weekly magazine after four or even six months, showing off a new postbaby "bikini body." Dear reader, it took me an entire year, thirteen months actually, to work off the weight I had gained in pregnancy. And that was just fine.

There were simply other things that were way more important to me, chief among them spending time with my daughter. But also trying to make things up to Teddy, and in general just finding a sense of normalcy again by putting the turmoil of the last twenty months behind us. I admit it was very hard not to feel depressed, insecure, and inferior. Stripped of my old figure, I had to get used to the new me. For a woman who had led my particular life, my body and its physical appearance were tied not only to my livelihood but to my womanhood and sense of worth. This is true for a lot of women, even those who don't work in front of the camera. Simply being born female in our society is to grow up being told your worth as a person is tied to how slim and attractive you are. Even for those of us lucky enough to have evolved parents, the message is still driven home by the world at large.

I had had the experience of being betrayed by my own womanhood because of endometriosis and the resulting lifetime of chronic pain, but then my womb had miraculously come through when no one thought it could. This gave me a new perspective on my body. My body had created this beautiful baby and was now sustaining her. For the first time in my life I consciously placed less value on how I looked. It just wasn't as important to me. I was profoundly thankful for what my body had produced.

In the span of just a few years, I had finally discovered what my condition was, struggled with the anger provoked by not having been diagnosed earlier, and then faced the sorrow of learning it was almost certain I couldn't have children. Wondering what would happen to my career if I couldn't lose the baby weight made me force myself to accept a reality I had not often considered. My looks were an asset I had consciously or unconsciously benefited from all my life.

When you have spent most of your adult life one way, and suddenly that changes, it's hard not to freak the hell out. And it's hard not to be distracted or worry about not meeting everyone's expectations, as well as your own, about an issue that is very central to many women's lives. So the only way I knew to not be distracted or disheartened by my weight gain was by making myself feel okay, good even, about my new size.

Making peace with myself about my body was the single most important thing I did to get my figure back. I just told myself that even if I did all the things I could to achieve my goals and I didn't get the expected result,

I would not feel bad about myself. I refused to let the shape of my body get me down. And that released me from the yoke I think all of us suffer under, whether postpregnancy or not. It freed me of the tyranny of my own mind and my self-judgments, all of which were based on an objectified view of who I was.

It worked. I actually began to love my body and wore clothes to show off my extra pounds and roundness. And when I talk about curves, I mean a double-F *poitrine*. And when I speak of being bigger, I mean going from a size 4 to a size 14. It was then that people started saying again how good I looked. I hadn't lost an ounce but I began to carry myself differently, move differently. I was really proud of my larger size, and enjoyed it. I began to feel womanly in a much earthier way. And I was much more brazenly confident than I had been when I had my usual slim figure. It was very weirdly exciting. I didn't suck in my belly and I didn't hide my size with clothing. I began to genuinely revel in my form. I threw away my newly bought postpregnancy Spanx (which I had hated with a passion all during filming the DC *Top Chef* promo shoot).

Because just as everybody is *not* meant to be a size 4, we all *are* meant to be different sizes at different times in our lives. We are meant to eat different things at different moments. Our needs shift as life shifts.

chapter 15

When Krishna was just about a year old, we went to film the *Top Chef* finale in the Bahamas. The whole crew was looking forward to getting away. It was still cold in New York City, where we were based. The winter had not yet given us any reprieve. We arrived at a huge, sprawling "family resort." This was not some tucked-away little beach village but a mini-city of various high-rises built in a semicircle configuration with swimming pools below and lounge chairs galore, leading all the way down to the shore, complete with bar and food service, DJs and lifeguards, pool activities and cabana boys. The resort had all the charm of a large white cruise ship, groaning with people, that goes nowhere. Off in the distance behind the towers you could see a large hybrid water slide–roller coaster. There was also an extensive aquarium in the main lobby, and many shops and restaurants.

Luckily, we were put in the building of time-share apartments rather than in the thick of the hotel. I didn't like the idea of Krishna eating hotel room service for so many days on end, so I made sure everywhere we stayed when traveling had a kitchen. I was looking forward to shooting, to let the baby have some sunshine. Adam came down to be with her. She was still nursing. It was and had been an awkward year.

The baby always went to see Adam in his New York hotel room, accompanied by my mom and our nanny, as well as a bodyguard. I felt compelled to have a private security officer follow Krishna when she went to see her father that first year. I had become afraid: of the press following us, which they did; of Adam deciding to do something drastic in the moment; and of my mother and the nanny being put in a vulnerable position. I wanted the women to have some support in that environment.

Adam became to me a completely unknown entity. I could not believe this was the same man who had built me the swing and accompanied me to India. But I wasn't going to make the mistake of misjudging things again, not when it came to my daughter or my mother. There wasn't much communication between me and Adam at all, and what was there was extremely fraught. I still felt very intimidated and threatened by him because of the incident in the hospital.

To be fair, Adam had e-mailed me and left voice messages, too, apologizing for his atrocious behavior. But now that I had seen that side of him, it frightened me to the core. It was the same fear and dread I had felt growing up, when Peter raised his voice or lost his temper. I wanted nothing to do with that kind of person. And I was worried, to say the least, that the baby would regularly be around someone capable of that kind of anger. I hadn't ever had a traditional relationship with Adam. We usually met for a date somewhere private, or hung out in a group with each other's very close friends or family for a finite period of only a few weeks at a time. We were never a regular couple, exposed to the trials and tests that committed couples face. I had no insight on how he handled stress or reacted to adversity. During the time I had known him, prior to my getting pregnant, he had only done everything to please me, or to present himself as a mild-mannered and even-tempered person. Now I had no idea with whom I was dealing, and Krishna and I were tied to him for the rest of our lives. We were all under strain, in a terrible pressure cooker of hurt feelings, fear, anger, and mutual resentment. I think the force of that pressure was too much for Adam, and he blew up. But some bells are hard to unring.

The effect of the blowup in the hospital would estrange Adam and me for the better part of the first four and a half years of Krishna's life. And the worst of that time was about to begin.

It was in the gorgeous and sunny Bahamas, with white sand and pleasant beaches filled with happy families on vacation, that I got word that Adam and I were about to go to war.

We were filming a lunch and then Judges' Table with several guest judges whom we had expressly flown in for the finale, like Morimoto and Michelle Bernstein, among others. The set was a glass-encased dining room in a building on one of the neighboring properties. The room was stifling, trapping the warm sun pouring in. I was sitting across from Wolfgang Puck. Suddenly, in the middle of asking for feedback from the other judges, I heard through my earpiece that we were stopping for a second. Then a producer stepped over to me on the set and quietly handed me her cell phone. She asked me to step away from the table. Because the next chef's food was about to be served, we took a very short break. I went outside into sunlight so violently bright, I could barely keep my eyes open.

My publicist, Christina, was on the line. She informed me that the *New York Post* and the New York *Daily News* had both phoned her separately. Both tabloids had in their possession a copy of a court filing submitted by plaintiff Adam Dell against defendant Padma Lakshmi. They asked if I had any comment on the lawsuit. I had no idea any such legal action had been filed. Immediately I felt faint, despite the large meal I had just consumed on the set. Christina said the documents seemed authentic. I put her on hold and called my attorney, who not only had handled my divorce quietly and quickly years prior, but had also been dealing with Adam's lawyer.

After Krishna's birth, the attorneys had drafted an agreement pertaining to visitation for the first year of Krishna's life that both Adam and I signed. Adam started agitating to negotiate a new one even before half the term of that first agreement had expired. The Dell lawyers had been threatening legal action for some time, repeatedly insinuating that I had far more to lose than Adam. I resented the implied threats to ruin my name and reputation, and thus my career, and they deepened my sense that Krishna's father was not to be trusted.

It would be another twenty-four hours before my attorneys received our copy of the filing. The rest of my conversation with Christina and my attorney seemed to take place in a fugue state. It would be the only time in twelve seasons of *Top Chef* that I went missing from my chair at Judges' Table. When I got back to my chair, Tom and Gail could see that the color in my face had drained. I had no choice but to continue with filming, but it was as if someone had turned down the volume on all of my senses. I couldn't walk off the set fast enough.

I was required to provide Adam with a weekly written report detailing every milestone or development in Krishna's life, including details about her diet and her daily activities. There were times I was, to be sure, way more descriptive than I needed to be. I liked writing about her, and tried to channel something born of strife into something positive: a journal of sorts Krishna could one day read of her early life.

June 18, 2010

KT spent this week in sunny California and had a ball. She was reunited with her grandmother and was very excited to see her again and listen to their personal made-up songs about fruit pies. She enjoyed hanging out at the pool but we were careful not to give her too much sun exposure as she is still too young even for sunblock. She has developed a light green ring around the pupils of her eyes so her baby blues may indeed be changing. Her eyebrows are also growing in and in spite of her fair hair is starting to look strikingly more Asian. She grows ever more beautiful and willful. She is enjoying herself.

July 30, 2010

This week was very eventful and exciting for KT. She arrived at her ancestral home in Madras to uncommonly cool weather and a warm welcome by her auntie Neela and her great-grandmother Jima. She had a couple of days of being cuddled and doted on and then went to Mumbai for two nights at the presidential suite at the Oberoi hotel where her mom had a photo shoot and every member of the staff promptly fell in love with her. She also experienced her first monsoon and had a lovely view of the Arabian Sea as torrential rains filtered the sunset over the bay outside her window. It was a very spooky and beautiful welcome and one that she took much glee in. She especially enjoyed her large bathtub but was overjoyed to return to her newly discovered bucket bath at her great-grandma's place. She also managed to turn on her side all by herself and then actually turn back. She pushes off her aunties' hands and inches forward to what looks like a mini crawling motion. She then gets tired and turns over. She also had her first taste of carrot, which she seemed to enjoy but then needed to be topped off by her mother's milk anyway. One has the sense that Krishna is very at home here. She is fascinated by her own face, as it now often sports a tiny jeweled bindi on her forehead. In fact, it gives her great pleasure to look at herself in the mirror and she is wondering why her mother insists on wrapping herself with this new type of dress but notes that the sari gives a greater sense of privacy and ease for breast-feeding. She has her own portable tent at all times.

December 12, 2010

Krishna is growing long and lovely. She is 29.5 inches and weighs 18.5 pounds. She is now able to stand by herself for 2 to 3 seconds before collapsing back down on her bum. She also learned how to clap her hands this week and give her loved ones a high five by slapping their hand. While she has an immense treasure trove of toys, *she prefers to play with her mother's silver coasters by knocking them off the coffee table and letting them clatter onto the floor, flinging them hither and yon. She loves lentils and rice with kale and cumin as well as mashed potatoes but has no palate for avocados whatsoever. She is pooping copious amounts.*

June 3, 2011

Krishna had a happy week. She is starting to remember passages to familiar songs she sings with various loved ones like "Row, Row, Row Your Boat" and "Lula-lu." She is also having a growth spurt and at times it seems she wakes up in the morning visibly bigger in size than when she went to bed just hours before. She also knows how to smile on cue for the camera and juts her face forward chin first. She has obtained possession of a much-coveted sable hair makeup brush and uses it to paint the cheeks of faces in her beloved magazines. She also rubs it across the back of her hand, enjoying the soft feathery bristles against her skin. The only blip was that she bumped her face quite hard into the wooden part of the bed at the beginning of this week and has a little bruise not only on her forehead but on her cheek as well. Those in her household are encouraging her to walk slowly rather than run but it seems our girl knows only one speed: full steam ahead.

I thought that by giving all this detail to Adam, especially since we were not speaking, I could show him that she was well cared for, and that Teddy and I were giving her a loving family life, even if it was not the traditional one he perhaps envisioned. But all this information only enraged him. He must have felt very left out. And so all his anger was harnessed in the contents of the court filing.

When I got to my hotel room, I was in shock. I couldn't believe Adam was suing me for full custody of our child. I couldn't imagine why he thought this was a good idea. My nanny, who had spent the afternoon with Adam and Krishna, knew about the lawsuit even before I did. Adam had had the "courtesy" to break the news to her just before he sent the two of them back to me. She was horrified and came home worried that I would be wrecked, unable to finish the shoot in the Bahamas. Luckily, by that time I had been hosting the show for quite a few seasons. I knew how to tune things out, or at least ignore my thoughts until I had time to fully process them. I just needed to get through the rest of the shoot, crown the next Top Chef, and go home. What made the experience particularly excruciating was that Adam was staying in the same hotel that we were. Over the next few days, some of the crew and executives actually bumped into him on the beach. He said cheerful hellos to them like nothing had happened, which made my colleagues deeply uncomfortable.

I called Teddy as soon as I reached my room and had fed Krishna. She was for some reason ravenous and wouldn't let go or stop suckling for a very long time. I did not want her near me when I spoke to Teddy, because I needed to vent out all my rage and sheer incredulousness at the stupidity of a public lawsuit. Who could be foolish and thoughtless enough to give the tabloids a court filing that contained the Social Security number of our child? Who could be such an idiot? And what father would think that this type of stress on the mother wouldn't bleed and affect a nursing infant?

When I phoned Teddy, he immediately said, "I know all about it, Junior." Jim Gallagher (the head of communications at IMG) had received a call from a friend of his at the Associated Press, who had a copy of the whole court filing on his desk already. It had been almost a year since Krishna was born, and more than that since we found out I was pregnant. In all that time, once I had made my decision to include Adam, Teddy had never once said, "I told you so." But now he really didn't know what else to say. He came down that weekend to give me moral support and even brought my assistant, Tucker, along on the plane for good measure. That Friday, when he arrived sometime in the early evening, I could only collapse into his arms and weep. "I tried to tell you . . ." He trailed off.

Teddy told me that of course he would try to be there for me as much as he could, but he really couldn't help things that much. "When I was in a position to help, Junior, you didn't take my advice." He said he knew my heart was in the right place, and that I was trying to do what was best for Krishna. "What you experienced with your old ex-husband is a picnic compared with what you're in for now. Just prepare yourself. Things are going to get very ugly, and I can't save you from this. You've got to face the storm. This is what you get for inviting this person into your bed, and into our lives."

It was very difficult to hear this, but Teddy was not a bullshitter. He would not soften the blow, because that would not have done me any good. We slept with the baby between us that night, hugging each other over her body. I felt like the world was about to crash over my head in the morning. I did not want the night to end.

The next morning I was to go back to work and he was going to play golf. Neither of us had slept very much, so as I went off to hair and makeup, and he said he wasn't feeling well, a bit tired and out of it, I didn't think much of it. He had had a hard week himself. Teddy decided to take it easy, to go to the beach or read the paper by the pool. That did seem a little odd to me—Teddy loved golf.

As soon as we landed back in New York there was a lot of work to catch up on with the jewelry company. And there was also a ton of planning and preparation for the lawsuit. The rest of January was a blur. I spent most of my energy trying to get our collection done for the buyers we had coming through the showroom in late February. February also meant the AT&T Pebble Beach National Pro-Am golf tournament, in which Teddy usually played. This year, he had asked his younger son, Everest, an excellent golfer, to take his place. Teddy seemed even more invested in the competition now that he was rooting for Everest, and even Judy—a dear friend and ex-girlfriend of Teddy's who had functioned as a mother of sorts to the boys—came with us to Northern California. Golf was something they did together, and they all loved it. I loved being there, and getting to see Judy was a treat, even if I personally did not know which end of the golf club was up. I was happy to be out of New York and to focus on Teddy and Everest and Krishna, leaving my troubles behind, if only temporarily.

I knew that, privately, Teddy was feeling bittersweet about bowing out of the tournament. But, he said, lately his swing just wasn't what it used to be—and he felt he hadn't had adequate time to practice. His swing had also become somewhat unpredictable. He could not control his shots as much as he felt he should've been able to, especially when he was normally a scratch player with a zero handicap. Teddy was hard on himself and had trouble accepting his limitations, but he was smart enough to know when he wasn't up to playing. So having Everest out on the green was a great plan. Secretly, selfishly, I wasn't upset about it at all. It gave Krishna and me a chance to spend more time with Teddy. I remember lying in the grass near the sea after breakfast, with him uncharacteristically joining us on the ground just looking up at the clouds. He had been slow to get up that morning. We lay there and Krishna sat on his stomach, and the three of us were just sunning ourselves in the chill early-spring air. "Isn't this better than walking miles and miles just to whack a ball with a stick?" I said jokingly. "I am not going to answer that," he said to me. Patting Krishna on the back, he said, "But Madam Junior, you understand that playing is better than watching any old day, right, kiddo?" He had taken to calling the baby "Madam Junior," or "Madam Squared" as a joke. Teddy got up then; he could never sit or lie still for long. I was struck by how he struggled to get on his feet. That was unlike him.

Later that day, when we were walking the course, with me pushing Krishna in her stroller as we followed Everest's progress, I noticed Teddy had trouble keeping his balance. He had almost tripped, over nothing, an invisible stone. When I went to help him, he pulled his arm away, saying he had just underslept and was tired—something he had been saying a lot lately.

I suppose I really didn't start to truly notice or worry about Teddy's health until that trip to Pebble Beach. Teddy was turning seventy-one that week. I had never been around a man that age who was as fit as Teddy. In fact, few men I had known, at any age, were as fit as Teddy. So when he started to slow down, I assumed it was the normal slowing down of someone in his stage of life. Also, he had come back from the African safari the year before with a case of spinal meningitis, or so it had been diagnosed. He had suffered terrible headaches ever since, and everyone kept saying it took a very long time to get over something like that. He was, after all, of a certain age.

But Judy hadn't seen him in a while, and she noticed the difference right away. From the moment she had boarded Teddy's plane in L.A., she had let him have it. "Teddy, hon, you don't look good," she'd drawled in her thick southern accent. "What the heck is wrong with you? Are you eating well? Padma, honey, are you keeping him out too late?" I could only point to Krishna, whom I was nursing under a blanket, a gesture meant to contain the whole of *Does it look like I've been having many nights out, with or without Teddy?* "Teddy, go see a doctor. Padma, drag him if you have to," she ordered.

I felt horrible that I hadn't noticed the severity of the change in him. But Teddy was proud and hated to seem weak in any way, and I am sure he hid many small signs from not only me, but also the world, just as he had tried to hide almost tripping on the sideline at Pebble Beach. We landed back in L.A. after the tournament. He and I spent the next two days in a specialist's office, as Teddy took test after test. He did every test his doctor could think of, and nothing turned up. I tried to celebrate his birthday by calling a few of his friends for a dinner at his house in Beverly Hills. In the end I called them all back to cancel. Teddy did not feel like company. He said he wanted only to be at home, alone together.

The next month he would, in frustration, check into the Mayo Clinic the minute they had an opening. There he would finally have an MRI, which Teddy had resisted getting because of his extreme claustrophobia. I offered to go to the Mayo Clinic with him, but he declined. He said I had too much going on, and he didn't want the baby dragged there. I think he was scared. I think he knew something was not right at all, and he didn't want me there to witness it with him. Teddy prided himself on seeming invincible to me, and as far as I was concerned, he *was* invincible. I tried to protest, but I was also aware of how compartmentalized Teddy's life was, even at the best of times. He had definite ideas about when and where he wanted to let people in. Having gone through a very intimate health crisis myself, I understood his need for privacy, and I respected it. But I did not like it just then. Teddy had always been there for me, even though perhaps I had not always deserved it. It was hard to let him go without me.

A few days later, my cell phone rang as I was boarding a flight to Florida, where I was headed to the Home Shopping Network to sell my Easy Exotic brand of culinary products. I saw that it was Teddy. I was struggling with the baby and the stroller, and getting both on the plane. So I called him back when we were settled into our seats. He was still at the Mayo Clinic. He said they'd found something in his head. The MRI had come back showing a mass around his brain. The doctors advised him that it could be an infection or something much worse. They referred him to a specialist surgeon at Sloan Kettering. I wanted desperately to get up with the baby and run off that plane. You did not get referred to Sloan Kettering unless there was a serious problem. They treated only one kind of malady there. Teddy told me to stay put. Suddenly, my little budding spice and tea business seemed trifling at best. I felt trapped by the plane's shutting door. "I will meet you in New York at the end of this weekend," I whispered into the phone. Tears streamed down my face, and I tried to turn toward Krishna in order to hide my face from the cabin crew standing right over me ready to demonstrate the safety procedures. Just weeks before, we had been in the Bahamas, and Teddy had been consoling *me* as I received what

I thought was my worst nightmare. Now I wished, with all my being, to be with him and confront together what actually *was* our worst nightmare. It seemed impossible. I spent the rest of the flight clutching Krishna to my chest and sobbing quietly under a blanket.

In early April, Teddy would have brain surgery at Sloan Kettering. He went to see a surgeon there named Dr. Gutin in the last days of March. Gutin explained that the mass could be a brain infection, a benign tumor sitting on his brain, or glioblastoma, the most serious form of brain cancer, for which there was no cure. Teddy said we needed to pray for a brain infection. He wanted to do the operation right away. He wanted to get it over with and get to the bottom of what was invading his head. The doctor said he would go in surgically and relieve pressure on the brain, but also remove anything he safely could that didn't belong there. I could understand Teddy's hurry, but my mother had by phone prepared me for what he might be like after the operation. I wanted just one more week, or month, or year, with Teddy and Krishna and me together. I wanted desperately to have a stretch of time that was calm, that was some form of normal, if only so we could taste what it felt like. I needed more time.

The September before, I had turned forty. On a hot, sweaty late-summer night we celebrated with much fanfare. The party, held at the restaurant Indochine, had a Toulouse-Lautrec theme, a marching band, and can-can girls traipsing through the restaurant. Among a sea of faces, many of whom he did not know, Teddy had toasted me. He spoke of how he thought I was "very capable, of doing whatever she sets out to do." I didn't feel capable at all at times. In fact, his unwavering belief in me outshone any real confidence I had in myself by a mile. But he was a great dreamer, a motivator, a doer, and a leader. As he toasted me, I found myself thinking about him, about the depth and indefatigability of his love and loyalty.

He was not my baby's father, but he loved her, more than life itself, provenance be damned. He was there when I delivered her. He was the first one to hold her. When they took turns waking each other up at night—she with her crying, he with his snoring—I laughed, exhausted and enraptured. She was not permitted to watch TV, but she was allowed to play at his feet when he watched hours of golf and tennis during those summer afternoons at the beach house when I deemed it too hot for her to play outside in the sun. That night, I had blown out the candles on my cake and wished for some harmony in our lives, to be able to simply love each other and have some laughs.

Everything had seemed so hard; even the good was mixed with strife and stress. The lawsuit only compounded that. But the news of something in Teddy's brain made all that had passed seem like child's play. Since Teddy's MRI, the lawsuit had turned into a menacing white noise. It hissed insistently in the background, following me everywhere, but I barely heard it now. It was a big stone in my shoe, but I kept walking. That was the terrible blessing of Teddy's health crisis: it had a shockingly clarifying power.

I woke up very early on April 5 and left the baby at home with the nanny. I traveled up the FDR by taxi, as I had done so many times, to meet Teddy at his home before accompanying him the few short blocks to Sloan Kettering. He had tried to keep me away, but I wouldn't agree. I think it was again because Teddy didn't want me to see him be afraid. He was always my rock, and still wanted to be. We were escorted to the pre-op room. It had the stale smell of rubbing alcohol and surgical tape. It was moderately crowded and humming already with uniformed nurses and surgeons milling about busily. Most of the other beds were occupied, with one or two people surrounding them. I remember thinking it was cold in there, and even felt the breeze coming down from an air-conditioning vent. The room was large and had several beds, each near a totem pole of stacked square computerized machines sprouting tubes that whizzed and whirred and lit up in sections, depending on who was hooked up to them. I could hear the hiss of a breathing machine. I heard a gurney traveling fast, far away down the hall.

I could tell by his body language that Teddy hated it here; he was physically irate. I pulled a thin white curtain around the bed to give him some privacy. He sat on the squishy hospital bed. The rubberized mattress beneath the cotton bedding squeaked under his weight. He removed his clothes, and as I folded them, he put on a wrinkled and flimsy cotton gown with ties in the back. He handed me the gold chain he wore around his neck and never took off. It had two gold Catholic pendants, and an oval tin one with Mary on it that I had given him. Mother Teresa had given it to me when I visited her in Calcutta years ago, and I had given it to him a couple of years back because it was the most precious thing I owned. When we pulled back the drape, the nurse suggested he wear the hospital-provided socks with slip guard strips, as the floor was slippery and not too clean, either. I kneeled down to put them on his feet. "Aww, jeez, would you getta load of *this* scene," he said, incredulous and looking down. "Hey, this is *exactly* the kind of thing I've been trying to avoid all along," I shot back. We both had a good laugh. I was glad to be there. I answered all the questions on the clipboard the nurse was holding, while another nurse started an IV on Teddy's arm.

During the surgery, I waited upstairs near his room with his sons for the doctor to call us down. I remember lying on a leather couch and dozing there long enough for my cheek to stick to the cushion. Two hours or so later, Margot, a woman from Teddy's office who was also waiting with the boys and me, came from the nurses' station and said Dr. Gutin had come out of surgery, and while they weren't finished with Teddy, he wanted to speak with us.

Dr. Gutin came into the small private room where we waited. It had pale-gray walls, wall-to-wall carpeting, and puce-colored faux leather and wood sofas. It was as bland and nondescript a room as possible, designed not to make any kind of impression on its occupants while they received potentially devastating news that would forever change their lives. There were four chairs facing each other, two on the left and two on the right. A couch was beyond them against the wall. Margot and Siya sat across from Everest and me. When he came in, the doctor still had on his OR scrubs and looked a bit sweaty and tired. He said that they had found the worst. The tumor had crossed the brain barrier to both lobes, and it was the deadliest of possibilities: glioblastoma. When I asked the doctor what that meant, he said "six to nine months or a year to live, maybe more if he has treatment; a year and a half if he's really lucky. But he must start treatment right away or he will be dead within six months."

It felt as if someone had inserted an electric rod into my side, and I wailed, an agonized, loud cry, like a wounded animal, a dog hit by a speeding car. I collapsed, weeping, into Everest's arms. I felt as if I were choking. I curled deeper into myself as my tears and snot stained his sleeve. My chest became concave with the sudden and sharp pain my body could not thwart. For everyone in the room, but especially for the boys, the moment was intense and agonizing. Love and respect dictate that I not speak to how Everest and Siya reacted to learning their father's fate, as it is not my story to tell for them. Such a private moment belongs to them alone.

Teddy had come back from Africa shortly before Krishna's birth not with spinal meningitis, but with this tumor. It had grown and developed just as the baby had. While Krishna learned to crawl on Teddy's plane, while she pulled herself up to stand and took her first steps, the tumor, too, had grown and taken root. While the baby grew each day, so did this invasion in his brain; this malignancy; this killer of joy, hope, of memory; this parasite.

I looked down at my watch, a simple Jaeger-LeCoultre Teddy had given me, a smaller replica of the one he wore. I saw it was 12:30 p.m. I had a meeting across Central Park, one of my very first with the overpriced court-appointed forensic specialist, Dr. Pizarro, whose job was to determine if I was psychologically fit to retain custody of my child and to report back to the court. As I walked to the elevator, I listened to a voice mail from Teddy I'd saved about the law suit after we flew back from the Bahamas. "Now, Junior, things are gonna get hard. You're going to have to keep calm, keep your head straight. You're smart, so be smart now. Don't get scared. This is real life. I will always be here, of course, but I can't always hold your hand. So prepare yourself." How was I going to prepare for what lay ahead? I could not even fathom what the future would look like.

Outside, on York Avenue, the trees were in bloom with tiny white flowers. Petals blew in the breeze like confetti. Thirty years earlier, I had routinely roller-skated to this very spot to meet my mother for her lunch break. We would buy two falafels, dripping with tahini and hot sauce, and eat together before she went back to her nursing shift. I thought of how Teddy would react to eating a falafel. "Ooof, sounds like a bellyache in a bag," he'd probably say. I hailed a cab and pushed my body inside. We headed across town. My mouth pronounced the address on the Upper West Side to the driver. The sound of my own voice was jarring to hear.

On my way to the psychiatric evaluation, I sat and blinked, motionless in the taxi. In one swift day, life as I knew it had changed. Again. What was waiting for me on the other side of the park would also have a great impact, on me and on Krishna, the only other person in my life as important as Teddy. I looked out the cab window and saw the sun come through the trees, light and shade dappling my face. We wended our way through spring in Central Park. The atmosphere was thick and I heard myself breathe. I could smell cut grass and cherry blossoms coming from the half-open car window. It was as if I had been dropped into some movie version of a life not mine, a melodrama that I, as a character, now had to assume was mine and resolve, a maze to which I did not know the end.

I knew that I had to get a hold of myself and put the life-altering information I had just received into the very back of my head until my meeting with Dr. Pizarro was over. I was advised by my attorneys not to cancel any appointments because it was important to be as reliable as possible. This one had been scheduled before Teddy's surgery and I just wanted to get on with it, get it out of the way. It would be better to do the interview when I was still in shock and on autopilot, before I had time to truly process what it all meant. The stakes were as serious as they could possibly be, so I had no choice but to put one foot in front of the other and walk into that office.

Dr. Pizarro was a very tall and broad-shouldered man. He had the same build and large body type as Adam, and he inspired the same uneasiness in me. I did not want to disrespect Teddy's privacy and so I withheld the gravity of the situation I had just come from. I told Pizarro that someone close to me had had surgery, to give context to any behavior of mine that seemed distracted or strange. I could not judge my words or movements accurately. My spirit went limp as I reentered my body, and I submitted myself to this man's questions, trying not to appear uninterested or dead inside. I answered him as concisely as I could. I asked if I could take notes, too, which I did in a small black Moleskine notebook I produced from my handbag. I tried to write down a few words that would jog my memory later when I recounted what had happened in the interview to my lawyers.

I felt like I was answering a compulsory questionnaire before I went to prison or my own execution. I had no choice but to be there. I didn't know if I could go up against the might of the Dell lawyers, and I could not go to Teddy for help. I didn't know how to process the information I'd just received from Dr. Gutin. I couldn't think. I did not have time to form any of my own opinions. I could only be present. I focused on what really mattered, Teddy and Krishna, and it somehow got me through the day.

In one instant, Dr. Gutin's news had given me great clarity. That was the terrible blessing again. I wanted to savor the love we had among the three of us; I wanted Teddy to feel as loved as possible every day he had left. I wanted Krishna to be shielded from the very real danger I constantly felt.

I didn't know what my life would look like or how much time I was going to have with the two people I loved most in the world. But I knew that if I could just get through this meeting, I could heave myself back into a taxi and go downtown, go home to nurse the baby in my arms, go home to grieve in private, go home to prepare for the worst.

chapter 16

By May, Teddy was well into chemo and radiation. I remember escorting him into the room where they keep the large cylindrical radiation machine. I had been in this very room thirty years ago when my mother had taken me to work one day. Unbelievably, the room had not changed at all in that time. I had the sense that I had stepped into the past, and I wished fervently for the power of time travel, to return to a time before Teddy was in pain, when the grim reality of this moment had been unthinkable. I would've given anything just to be able to slow down time at least a little. But of course I couldn't. So when I first received the schedule for the next season of *Top Chef*—filming would resume at the end of June and go through early August—I thought seriously of bowing out. Teddy did not want me to stop working. I felt tremendously conflicted, but Teddy insisted.

I flew home twice during filming that summer, and each time Teddy seemed thinner and thinner. We spent the remainder of August shuttling back and forth between his beach house in the Hamptons, where we spent the weekends, and the city, where during the week he had chemo and radiation at Sloan Kettering.

We were all happier and less stressed at the beach. Teddy played well with Krishna, and she relished his attention. She made him laugh to no end, and they seemed to have their own language and private conversations. Teddy had always been more physical with the baby than I was, and she did not understand why her poppy was now so standoffish. She was much more verbal by this time and would try to pull Teddy physically toward the swimming pool.

Just a summer before, he had spent most weekends teaching her how to float and swim, supporting her little body with one open hand. She would also sit upright on the couch next to him in the TV room, amused during golf or tennis matches, cooing and smiling at his commentary. "Aw jeez, would you getta loada *that* swing, for crying out loud," he'd complain to his pint-sized sidekick while she shook her sippy cup in agreement. This was the only time Krishna got to watch TV, and she was *mesmerized* by any person swinging any blunt object at some ball or other on the screen. "You'd never choke like that, right, kiddo? No can doosky!" I would pop my head in every now and then from the kitchen to see what they were up to, and they were as content as two peas in a pod.

This summer, however, Krishna was not only more verbal but also very mobile, and she was getting heavier. She would climb all over Teddy until one of his sons would come and lift her off him. She tugged at her poppy's sleeve, begging him to take her out. When he said he couldn't, she climbed onto the couch and went directly for his head. She gently stroked the ropy, livid J-shaped scar on the side of his scalp. "You boo-boo? Is okay, is okay, Poppy better," she soothed, mimicking the voice I would use when she fell, bumping her elbow or scraping her knee. Those last days of summer, not only did Krishna have growth spurts but her language skills, too, developed rapidly. It felt to me that with every leap forward I sensed in her, Teddy took a turn for the worse.

On one of my trips home during filming, Teddy had become extremely dehydrated and I drove him to the Southampton hospital, where we met a tall and sturdy nurse named Sarah in the ER. I asked her if she ever did private duty and she said yes. The advent of Sarah in our daily lives at the beach was both a blessing and the curse of the inevitable. Krishna was at first scared of this big woman dressed in white who seemed to always want to prick her poppy with needles and tubes. But eventually, Krishna got familiar with Sarah, and the IV pole, too, helping to push it alongside her poppy as he struggled to stay on his feet long enough to get from couch to dining room. It frightened me to see Teddy's physical strength ebb away from him. He had always been a solid and strong presence, virile and active, even when compared with men younger than him, whose hair was nowhere as thick as the shock of white he trimmed twice every month. His posture began to suffer and we all struggled to get him to eat enough.

We were losing him.

Watching Siya or Everest help Teddy walk, Krishna wanted to help, too. This ragtag procession broke my heart but was at times also comical as we tried both to keep Krishna out of the way and to let her feel a part of all the activity. Everest was the preferred choice for Teddy to lean on, and so Siya and I usually trailed slightly behind, steadying the IV pole and hoping neither Teddy nor Krishna would trip or fall over each other.

One early evening, I looked outside at the tall, reedy grass growing between the house and the ocean. The sun was setting. The already tan stalks glowed golden in the last light of the day, and I could hear the sea over the television. The tall shrubs swayed and rubbed against one another, rustling in the sea wind. The wet aroma of tomatoes simmering in the kitchen hung in the air like a warm cloak. Maggie, Teddy's cook, was stewing up a cauldron of the last of the late-summer tomatoes. My stomach grumbled. Now and then I could hear a yelp or a whoop from the front of the house, where Everest and Siya were playing tennis. The baby played at our feet with some blocks.

Teddy said he had just been remembering a dinner we had attended together, but that the memory didn't make sense. He didn't know why. He didn't know what he was saying exactly, but he knew enough to know that his brain was playing tricks on him. It worried him. He thought that what he remembered happening hadn't happened. He was right. The memory was a jumble of memories conflated into one. He had overlapped separate events and did not know how to untangle them. He didn't know what was true and what was his mind short-circuiting. He said there had been a dinner or a big banquet, and it looked like I was shooting *Top Chef*, but he was there, too. And for some reason the chef Daniel Boulud was with us.

All three things he remembered were a plausible combination. Teddy did throw a big charity dinner around that time every year called Huggy Bear. But this was not a Huggy Bear dinner, he said. And he knew Daniel well, too. Teddy dined often at Café Boulud, which was coincidentally in the lobby of the Surrey Hotel, for years with his mother and then with me. We dined at the restaurant Daniel on special occasions, too. I had arranged his seventieth-birthday dinner there, a week before Krishna was born. Teddy loved the steak and when he got too sick to eat out, Daniel sweetly sent rib eye and potatoes home to the Manhattan apartment with the driver. Teddy had also visited me on the set many times, but never for a big event or banquet. He knew all this, but he still had trouble sorting through what was real and what was imagined. The confusion. He could not tell the subtle but important difference between possibility and actual memory. That was the first time he noticed being confused. It scared us both. Losing his mental faculties was his worst nightmare.

I felt the evening chill creep into me and reached for a nearby blanket. "Summer is almost over," I said, trying to change the subject. "So am I," his eyes seemed to be saying back.

Sometime after my forty-first birthday on September 1, back in the city, I was still trying to jump-start Teddy's appetite. I wrapped Krishna up into my Baby Bjorn (although she was getting heavy by this time) and went to the farmers' market in Union Square hunting for goodies. A trip to the Greenmarket always gave me a sense of well-being and elevated my mood. It was a favorite outing for Krishna, too. She loved all the hustle and bustle of the vendors and the motley crowd that passed through; the dreadlocked skateboarders whizzing by; the flowers she stuck her nose right into on days we went with the stroller; and the piles and piles of fruits, vegetables, cheeses, and breads and other baked treats heaped in every stall. It was my favorite time of year, the hinge moment between seasons, between the full bloom of summer and the chill of fall creeping in slowly.

Krishna enjoyed touching and fingering all the different-colored vegetables like spiky, spiraled neon-green Romanesco; yellow and purple corn, with their soft silk sprouting at the top; nubby sweet potatoes; fuzzy peaches; and juicy plums. She ate blueberries by the handful, and loved the crisp bite of sliced Asian pear. And she was a good sport about trying every strange nugget of cheese that was offered. All the vendors were more than generous with their samples, waving them in front of her nose. She dangled from my torso facing outward, eager to taste the world she had yet to discover. The market was exhilarating, a bountiful place to exercise her senses.

The chemo made Teddy quite debilitated and nauseous, and the thrush that came with it coated his taste buds like a blanket of snow covering spring grass. Even the Marinol pills did little to restore his interest in food. Teddy's appetite had been decreasing by the day, and I could think of nothing as nourishing as a white ragu made with veal and mushrooms that he loved. He had eaten a similar version almost weekly across the street from his office at Cipriani, in the Sherry-Netherland hotel. I found some lovely hen-of-the-woods mushrooms, and some trumpets, too. I bought fresh dill and other tender herbs from my favorite stall, which also had at this time what I considered to be the jewels of the farmers' market: chili peppers.

Hot, and hotter, and hottest chili peppers, in bright red, dark green, marigold yellow, and purple-black as well as a fluorescent orange. All spring and well into the end of summer, this stall was one of the biggest in the market, consisting of a horseshoe of three tables with lanes of tables in the middle. Behind the back wall of tables, hanging from the tent covering, was a chart listing the different kinds of peppers and their supposed numerical rating on the Scoville scale. This stall, laden with these riches, was what I looked forward to most. I disregarded the famous measurer of capsaicin (the substance that provides spicy heat) in each of the peppers and preferred to sample them on my own, usually with a bit of bread and cheese in hand to quell the sting between bites. I bought a handful of Scotch bonnets, about a cup of green and red small Thai chilies for cooking, and a heavy cellophane bag of round red cherry peppers the size of Ping-Pong balls. I always bought a random sampling of ones I was curious about, mostly for their physical beauty. I made sure to get a decent-sized bag of mild chilies for Krishna's sake. She could not resist getting in on the action. I had to fend off her arms, outstretched inside mine, trying to touch every colorful and dangerous little bomb as I bent forward. I usually made her hold the hunk of bread, and she would gnaw on it, soaking it with her saliva.

These peppers were not for Teddy. He never liked his food very spicy, even at his healthiest. These peppers were not for Krishna. Most were way too hot, even if she did eat much spicier food than others her age. These peppers were for me, shiny and ready to unleash their power into some otherwise bland dish. One of my favorite pastimes was to bring home a big haul of different peppers and experiment, making up new chutneys or blending them with fruits like green apple or hard green plums for a sweet and sour relish. My mother has always been the condiment queen of our family, whipping up sauces in her blender or with her mortar and pestle, with magic in her hands. She could turn any boring lunch or dinner into an intensely tantalizing experience of hot and sweet and sour flavors exploding in your mouth at once, by just adding a sauce or relish on the side. I had inherited the same itch, if not yet honed a subtlety of palate like hers. I liked the jagged spike of fresh salsas, and the mellow depth of slow-cooked chutneys, too.

But in those days what I was most interested in was pickling. I had been around the grand ritual of pickle making when I was young, of course, in my grandmother's home. And when we first moved to Los Angeles and stayed with my uncle Bharat, my mother made many pickles with the citrus in their backyard. But those were Indian pickles. They were very complicated to make and often perfumed up the house for days with the aroma of mustard oil and frying spices. Some Indian pickles have a laundry list of ingredients that runs for miles, including many you could never even taste anyway. My foremothers assured me that every ingredient was essential, whether I knew why or not, and considering the heat of the chilies involved, nothing should be omitted because you needed these ingredients to buffer the stomach. Regardless, all that alchemy and the array of items to achieve it were not in the cards at that strange juncture of my life. What I got very interested in was simple preservation.

Pickling is a great activity. It requires very few ingredients besides the vegetable you are actually pickling. A handful of seeds, herbs, and twigs thrown into salted vinegar and you are in business. Simply submerging your favorite summer vegetables or early fall chilies in liquid and seasonings takes mere minutes, and bestows months of good bottled heat in the dead of winter.

Krishna immediately fell in love with pickling. Pickles were the first thing we made together. She had seen me add pickled chili peppers to countless dishes. She was fascinated by the ceremony of it. We filled the lids of spice bottles with coriander seeds, oregano, and black peppercorns, arranging them in an assembly line on the counter. Then I poured clear vinegar into a large pickling jar, adding enough salt and a spoonful of sugar. It delighted her to see these dissolve, disappearing with every stir of her wooden spoon like magic. She tried to not stir too swiftly while I coarsely sliced some onions and

krishna's pickled peppers

Makes a dozen pickled peppers

2½ cups distilled white vinegar

¾ teaspoon kosher salt

¼ teaspoon granulated sugar

1 medium carrot (2 to 3 ounces), cut into ¼-inch-thick slices on the
   bias

½ small yellow onion (2 to 3 ounces), cut into ¼-inch-thick crescents

12 medium fresh jalapeños or other chili peppers (approximately 14
   ounces)

½ teaspoon whole coriander seed

1 teaspoon Mexican oregano

In a measuring cup, mix the vinegar, salt, and sugar until completely
dissolved. Set aside.

In a large bowl, combine the carrot, onion, jalapeños, coriander
seed, and oregano. Toss together with your hands to mix evenly.

Fill a 1-liter glass jar with the spiced vegetables, taking care to
scrape any remaining spices from the bowl to the jar. Carefully pour
the vinegar mixture into the jar, pressing the vegetables down with a
wooden spoon if needed.

Cover the jar with an airtight lid. The pickled peppers will be ready
to enjoy in 2 to 3 months.

carrots on the bias. We added the spices to the jar one by one. She loved to watch them swirl around, sticking her little fingers into the vinegar to taste. We tossed the cherry peppers with the other vegetables into a bowl, and she mixed them with her hands. While I tried to gently plop them into the jar, she laughed, plunging her whole hand into the cold, salty vinegar.

There was so much tactile pleasure in pickle making, and little she couldn't participate in. It gave her a deep sense of pride to display the bottles on our counter, which was right opposite the front door. Whenever a new person entered the house, she would indicate that she had made them herself by running over to where they were and pointing upward, saying, "Look my pickles! I made pickles!" She kept asking when they would be ready, the glowing red orbs in ever amber-colored water. That they were most likely too hot and she would never be able to eat them herself did not curtail her suspense and anticipation. I kept telling her they wouldn't be ready for months, because at first she would look at them every day, shaking them at the base with both hands in such a way I feared they would slide off and come crashing down over her head. "When, Momma, when?" "When it gets really cold, and you wear the heavy coat for the snow," I said. It occurred to me then that by the time I took my first bite of these pickles, so lovingly made and impatiently waited for by Krishna, Teddy might not be around. I wanted the next days to go slowly as much as Krishna wanted them to speed up. Outside our window, I saw the first leaf fall from the maple tree, turning and swirling hopelessly toward its death on the ground below.

It was almost Halloween. Krishna was a lion. She had a costume that looked exactly like a child-sized replica of the Cowardly Lion in *The Wizard of Oz*. It was the perfect costume, furry and soft and warm. Her rosy cheeks and dimpled chin smiled from ear to ear with self-satisfaction. Teddy had been sleeping a lot that weekend since we got to the house on Meadow Lane.

He hadn't been up at all since going to bed early the evening before, but he could feel me in the bed with him. He held and squeezed my hand when I slipped it into his. He interlaced his fingers with mine. He was pretty weak then. He had to use the wheelchair at all times, and he hated it. And he was thin. So very thin. When I turned to hug him, pressing my body up against his back, I could feel his ribs on my breasts, the bones of his arm and shoulder, even his tailbone and pelvis against my front.

Krishna and I had gone apple picking with Maggie down Route 27, and I was making applesauce for her and Teddy, with lots and lots of cinnamon and butter. Teddy loved cinnamon; he had it in his coffee every day. But he no longer drank coffee. When the thrush and chemo made his throat sore, it became hard for him to swallow. He began to choke on simple soft roast chicken. He just couldn't be bothered to chew, either. But I knew he loved my applesauce. It was warm and wet, and sweet. It would go down, if anything could. Krishna loved it, too. It was her favorite, neck and neck with Tha-Tha's banana *payasam*. The house smelled of brown butter and cinnamon and stewed apples. There was enough so that Maggie and I put some in containers to cool on the counter. And even a portion for us to take back to the city. There was a definite chill already and the autumn leaves were rustling in the wind from the sea. None of us had walked on the beach for quite a while. It was too cold. I hoped what had been bubbling on the stove would keep us all warm.

Judy was there, too. Judy doted on Krishna, and Krishna loved her. They even shared the same birthday. And they had similar dispositions. Judy had brought Krishna a set of fairy wings that were delicate, gauzy, and pink, with a wand and crown, and they delighted Krishna. I also got her a mail-order white tiger costume, which was for indoors. We had just seen a live white tiger at the Ringling Bros. circus also named Krishna, while I was filming the show in Texas that summer, so she had wanted to be that for Halloween. But I couldn't resist getting the lion. It would keep her warm on its own if she went trick-or-treating outdoors. She looked fantastic in all of them.

The late-afternoon sun was getting low. Krishna wanted to show her poppy her Halloween getup, and she wouldn't accept that he could not be awakened to look at it. The bed was almost as tall as she was, but she had recently learned to wedge her toes deep into the crevice between the box spring and the mattress to hoist herself up. She sometimes pulled on a sheet for leverage, though at times she pulled on Teddy. I walked in and saw this small brown animal creep up and startle poor Teddy, who let out a low groan. "Poppy, wake up. Wake *up* now, Poppy!" She had been waiting patiently way past lunch and now she couldn't stand it any longer. I was afraid she would hurt him or herself. I came up from behind and carried her up into the bed. I told her to be very careful because Poppy wasn't feeling strong. Teddy had some random purplish bruises on his forearm from all the treatments and I pointed them out to Krishna, to always be careful where she grabbed Poppy. She was so used to being rough with him, to just climbing all over him at will. I put her carefully on my side of the bed next to him. He happened to be turned inward toward where I would sleep. She was as careful as it's possible for a toddler under two to be. I was moved by how her little hand rubbed his forearm. She put her face right up close to his, as much as the woolly mane would allow her to. "Poppy, wake up! Look, I'm a lion."

I lay down on the other side of Krishna to make sure I could buffer any sudden movements she made. The remaining hair that was not shaved off on the side of Teddy's head had been shorn to a very short quarter-inch of salt-and-pepper stubble. And it made him look strangely like a little boy sleeping with his hands under his stubbled chin. He did not open his eyes. "Mmm," he moaned, clearly disturbed. "Poppy, I'm a scary lion, *arrg!*" Her poppy was not getting up. "Poppy, Poppy, get up!" She squealed right into his face. "Let him sleep, *kanna.*" I tried to gently pull her away by the waist. "Just open your eyes," she cajoled. "Open. *Poppy.* See?"

I didn't know then that it would be the last exchange between Krishna and her poppy, but what I saw scared me. "Hey, if you can hear us, Teddy, blink," I said quietly. He did not blink. But then the corner of his mouth turned up ever so slightly. And then he slowly opened his eyes and shut them again rapidly, as if to say, "Not there yet, Junior." Without opening them again, he said, "Hey, kiddo." Now Krishna became emboldened and lunged her face back closer to his. "Look! I'm a lion." "You are a lion." "You're not looking," she accused. Teddy with great effort opened his eyes again. They stared at each other for what seemed like a long time. All I could hear was Teddy's breathing, slow and heavy. Krishna couldn't stand the silence. "I love you, Poppy. Oh yes. I. Do." Teddy closed his eyes. "I love you, too, kiddo. Have fun."

Before he could finish, she was already scrambling down to the wooden bench at the foot of the bed. From there she could make it to the ground easily. She scampered off to find Judy or Maggie. I stayed there for a few minutes. I moved closer to Teddy and tried to put my arm around his waist, but after a few seconds felt the weight of my arm was too much on his torso. "You okay?" I asked him. "Yeah, just tired. She's a lion." That night would be the last night Teddy and I would sleep in that house together. Or share any bed again.

It was very early in the morning of November 20 when the call came. So early that it was still dark in the bedroom, with not even a sliver of light peeking through the space between wall and window shade. Krishna shifted slightly at the first ring, but the soft rumble of her nostrils did not break the sleepy rhythm of light snoring. She had woken up a few hours before, crying out. I managed to pat her back to sleep. I thought then that she'd had a bad dream. By the second ring, I was out of bed. When I got to the phone, charging in the kitchen, the ringing had stopped. Bleary-eyed but awake, somehow I knew. He was no more.

The night had been uneasy from the start. After a supper of peas, carrots, shrimp, and rice noodles, Krishna and I got into the bath later than usual. I could feel her bum bouncing on my thigh as I soaped her neck and shoulders. Along with the yellow duckies and other tub toys, a few noodles and peas bobbed in the soapy water, stowaways in the many folds of her belly. I washed her hair with one hand as I fished for the stray pea, the odd noodle, with the other. I ladled water over her head with a plastic mug. As I washed her, an alarm began to ring in my head, faint at first, then louder and louder.

I felt fingers scratch at my torso. I looked down to see my heartbeat pulsing visibly, wildly, and her open mouth reaching for a nipple. I parried her attempt, guiding her lips away. "I want . . . ," she whimpered. I had already weaned her, but she still wanted her way. I needed to find my phone. "No more Mommy's milk, *kanna*," I said, spinning her slippery frame to face forward, then pulling the drain. I got out of the bath and reached for my phone. My hand dripping and now shaking, I dialed his home. Cursorily wrapped in a towel, I stood in the doorway, watching her in the tub.

"Hi, Padma." His housekeeper, Sandy, answered before I'd spoken. My throat tight, I asked if everything was okay, if I should just bundle the baby up and come over. A cab, the FDR, I could be there in ten minutes. Something was wrong. I could feel it. "They're up there with him," she said, referring to his siblings, who had by then come in and taken over his care in the last stages of his illness. "Let me check." I had dressed by the time I heard Sandy's voice again. Water from my hair dripped down my spine beneath my sweater. I kept my eye trained on Krishna's glistening back as she sat in the now-empty tub with her toys strewn around her, humming softly and coloring with bath crayons on her newly enlarged canvas. Two ducks, run aground, were nestled against her lower back, beak to beak as if kissing. *How strange this looks,* I thought, *how arranged.*

"They said to tell you there's no change." I had known Sandy for more than four years by then and could tell how tired she was by the strain in her Bosnian accent. The next time Sandy and I would speak would be at the Frank E. Campbell Funeral Home.

Early that next morning, after I'd felt my way in the dark to the phone, I saw who had called. I took the phone to the living room and sat down on the green velvet couch. I dialed his sister's number for confirmation, though I needed none. She wouldn't tell me the exact time of death. But I knew when in the middle of the night he had chosen to go. Even the baby had; it seemed she had woken up to say good-bye. I couldn't go back into the bedroom. I couldn't bear to lie down next to her, my body now filled with this irrevocable information. I wanted her to continue sleeping in a world that still contained her poppy, for as long as she could.

For months I had known this day would come. From the moment seven and a half months prior when the surgeon, still in his scrubs, had told me and Teddy's children of the large, voracious tumor in his brain. Throughout the sweet heartbreak of watching Krishna learn the names of his nurses, seeing her gradually grasp the purpose of the IV they tended, which, as she put it, was meant to cure "the big boo-boo in Poppy's head." Still, despite my almost daily rehearsal of the inevitable, the event itself, the blow to the gut, was no less startling than if his plane had fallen out of the sky. When I heard the news, for a moment I saw my life without him, the many lonely years ahead of me. I sat motionless until a wave of grief toppled me sideways and my tears soaked the couch. Sometime later, dawn broke over the East River, and the living room glowed with gentle light. My heaving sobs and tears had stopped. I lay there, very still, until the bedroom door clicked open. Krishna shuffled out and stopped, blinking. "Mommy, I'm scared," she said, the first time she had ever used that word. I stood up, took her in my arms, and held her, thinking but never saying, *me too.*

I ached for him now, for his "dashing man" smell, for his booming voice as he called out to me as I primped in front of the mirror: "Hurry up now, Junior, we haven't got all day." Indeed, we hadn't had enough time at all.

applesauce for teddy

10 medium mixed apples (approximately 3 pounds), cored, peeled,
    and cut into 16 pieces each
Juice of 1 medium-sized lemon (approximately 2 tablespoons)
½ cup (1 stick) unsalted butter
½ cup cane sugar
¼ teaspoon kosher salt
1½ tablespoons ground cinnamon
¼ teaspoon ground clove

Put the apples into a bowl and toss them with the lemon juice.

In a deep pot, melt the butter over medium-low heat. Once the butter is evenly melted and slightly brown, add the apples with their juices and stir. Cook for 1 minute.

Add the sugar, salt, cinnamon, and cloves, sprinkling evenly throughout, and stir vigorously to distribute.

Raise the heat to medium and cover. Cook covered for approximately 25 to 30 minutes, depending on how chunky you like your applesauce. You'll need to cook longer for smoother applesauce. Every 5 minutes, uncover and stir briskly, breaking up the chunks of apple with the side of your spoon, then replace the lid.

Serve warm.

chapter 17

The world had changed. It had dimmed. It was as if my eyes had been traded for some other lenses, ones with a darker filter through which less light got through. I was fine with this. I wrapped my grief around me like a cloak. I took comfort in it. I went out into the sunlight of the outside world only when my work or Krishna required it. I focused on just three things: Krishna, work, and Teddy's being gone. He had entered my life and in so doing had altered it completely and ineradicably, and now his death, his exit, altered it anew. My cocoon of grief became so familiar to me, so safe, so cozy, that I did not *want* to venture out. This is how life will be, I thought.

In January 2012, less than two months after Teddy's death, I would enter the Supreme Court of the State of New York for the first day of the custody trial. I was on autopilot. There were opening statements. A couple of observers sat in the back of the courtroom listening. And then I took the stand. I remember thinking how shiny Adam's shoes looked, how big his feet appeared under the table he sat at with his lawyers. My attorneys had prepared me by instructing me to be concise in my answers and to tell the truth. *Answer only the question asked of you. Do not get rattled by the other side,* they had warned. I felt as if nothing could rattle me again. After two hours of questioning, we broke for lunch. The Dell lawyers had done their best to find some fault with my parenting in their opening statement and realized they could not after I took the stand. And so Adam's side asked for a recess over the weekend to negotiate out of court. I was never cross-examined. And Adam would not take the stand. By that Monday, we reached a settlement. I walked away numb but with no significant change to what was in place before the litigation. In the end, Krishna's last name would be hyphenated to include Adam's surname. She would now be called Krishna Thea Lakshmi-Dell, a small price to pay for an end to the meaningless and expensive anguish.

That March, Krishna and I went to the Hamptons house for the last time to say good-bye to the place the three of us had been happiest and to bring home what tangible memories we could. I bent down in the driveway and filled a ziplock bag with the pebbles he drove over by the tennis courts. I wanted anything he had touched: the cracked wood canister by his bedside that held his pens and pencils, the clay bowl in our dressing room he threw his golf gloves and extra tees into when he came home. I had coveted his comb, and the Guerlain cologne and deodorant that Maggie had rescued for me from his medicine cabinet right after his death. I could not stop the voracious appetite I had for my lover's things and they somehow had magnified meaning now, because I could not find meaning in his being gone.

The year or so that followed Teddy's passing I spent in a walking daze, focusing on Krishna and her ever-changing needs. My friends and family came together around us and did their best to comfort me and keep me busy. But mostly I was engulfed in my own private universe, going to work when required, and otherwise just being with Krishna. She was great company, and succor to my grief. She also slept with me, just as I had slept with Neela back in India. This gave me an enormous sense of physical well-being. I didn't date, couldn't imagine or consider it really. I didn't feel like I was single, just that my lover happened to be dead. Two years on, I still felt like Teddy was with me.

Krishna was my sole source of bodily contact, and that was more than fine. I couldn't fathom having any man close to me, and I returned to an almost childlike, prepubescent state. My sexuality was nonexistent, and that was actually liberating. On the weekends when Krishna went to Adam's, I relished being alone, rattling around the house talking out loud to Teddy like some crazy old lady, and luxuriating in the peace and quiet. So much had happened that I was psychically exhausted. I couldn't reenter life as others knew it, but I was trying.

When Neela told me her younger daughter, Akshara, was getting married, I knew I had to find the wherewithal to push through my self-imposed hermitism. The wedding would be on Valentine's Day 2013. February 14 has always been a special day in our family. It was Neela's birthday. This year she would turn fifty. It was also the day after Teddy's birthday, so it had become dark for me after he died. I was happy that it would now represent another joyous occasion, a new beginning for Akshara and Ravi, her husband-to-be. In our family, we call each other not only on birthdays, but also on anniversaries. I was happy to add the date to my calendar, knowing that from then on, I'd have yet another reason to express my love to the people who meant the most to me.

India was the perfect salve to my wounds. Krishna was a great traveler. Over the few short years of her life, she had clocked more miles than most adults. Her disposition was easy and pleasant, and she had the uncanny ability to amuse herself on planes while I dozed and read. It was astonishing. She had been to Chennai before, but this would be the first time she'd actually remember it.

We arrived from New York after a daylong slog through airports and planes and traffic. It was 10:00 p.m. local time, but my body had no idea if it was night or day. Krishna was hungry, so I found some left-over *dosa* batter in the kitchen and started making one for her. Next thing I knew, my grandmother was by my side, commandeering the griddle. "Let me do it," she said. "You don't know where anything is." I insisted, but she won, even though by then she cooked with only one arm, the other still paralyzed from the stroke. Then my aunt Papu came in and yelped, "You're making your grandma cook?" She was appalled. "It's ten at night!" Papu took over, my grandmother wouldn't leave, and my uncle Ravi entered the fray. "Look at you," he said. "You're supposed to be this famous food person and you're making these women cook at ten o'clock!" I quickly remembered how it felt to live with so many people. Every move you make is scrutinized. You get up and it's "Where are you going?" You come back and it's "Why are you wearing that blouse? I like the other one better." You walk outside and someone calls from the veranda, "Don't go *that* way, there's too much sun!" It was exasperating and suffocating and God, I had *missed* it.

The year before, my success had allowed me to move Neela and my grandmother out of our childhood home to a larger, newer place. By my calculations, I still owed them much more. This larger three-bedroom apartment, still in Besant Nagar but on a quieter, tree-lined street, had a night watchman at the entrance of the complex. Not only did I want to be more comfortable whenever I visited, but the old flat in Besant Nagar, which was to become the site of Neela's sari-and-blouse-making operation, needed repairs. The plumbing, electrical wiring, kitchen, and bathrooms in that house were much the same as when I was in third grade.

The city of Chennai itself, however, was much different from what it was when I had built sand temples in the courtyard. The city that had felt in many ways like a sleepy town had become a frenetic metropolis. Much of the sand was now asphalt. St. Michael's Academy had expanded into a large compound with tall buildings and fields for soccer and cricket. The

Milk Bar that was once a leafy oasis was now a seedy, dilapidated place to be avoided.

Neela and I visited the old flat. All around our old building, urban development now made the area feel very congested. We could no longer see the ocean from my grandfather's bedroom window. Taller buildings had been erected all around. Everyone wanted to live near the sea. The courtyard below had been asphalted, too. Children no longer made temples in the sand. I couldn't believe how small the flat looked. It had always felt huge to me. I visited each room, could still see the lizards where the cracked walls met the ceiling. The place was empty save for some sewing machines and tailors, employees of Neela's business. So many of us had grown up here, fought as children here, cried as teenagers, and often run back to this place as adults. Several sewing machines hummed as I walked barefoot on the old green marble from room to room. Underneath the hum, I could still hear echoes of Rajni tattling on me to Bhanu, the screech of my grandfather's metal desk chair as he rose to say good-bye to a student. The house had never been beautiful, but it was beautiful to me, even in its dilapidated and empty state.

Yet for all the changes, much felt the same in the new apartment. There were still buckets of hot water for bathing, in spite of showerheads being installed in these new bathrooms. There were still far too many of us, old and young, from my grandmother to Krishna. We would crowd onto the floor, draping ourselves on pillows, grooming and feeding like a troop of monkeys, me scratching my nephew Sidhanth's back, Neela braiding my hair, kids climbing among our bodies. Aunt Bhanu kneeling on the floor, peeling potatoes or mangoes. My grandmother haggling with every vendor she came across on the porch below.

And we still talked, a lot. Our conversations were a blur of languages. Everyone in the household was tri- or even quadrilingual. I grew up speaking Tamil, the language of my ethnicity; Hindi, the national language but also the language of Delhi; and English. Others in my family added Malayalam, the language of Kerala, my ancestral home, to that list. "Please" and "okay" were in English and bookended many bursts of speech. "Please"—someone might begin, then switch to Hindi—"could you make some chai for me?" Then, without skipping a beat, she might continue in Tamil, "I'm really craving it"—then back to English—"Okay?" Certain words were just better in one language than another.

And still, just as soon as the plates from lunch were cleared, we talked about what we might have for dinner. When tiffin time came, my grandmother and Neela still disappeared into the kitchen to short-order-cook *dosa*, bringing them to us as they were ready, our greed and impatience scorching our fingers as we tore apart the crepes. We still walked on Elliot's Beach, and as we turned back toward home, we still had to make the old heart-wrenching decision whether to stay in for dinner or go out for *chaat*.

The new place had cool marble floors, too, though not speckled green but glossy beige. Each bedroom had its own veranda and bathroom: one for my grandma, one for Neela, and one for Krishna and me when we came. Still, because of the wedding, we managed to fill every square inch of floor with out-of-town relatives. As lovely as Krishna had been on the plane, she was now in as foul a mood. At home in the East Village, it was usually just the two of us. My mother and Peter came to visit once every other month. Here, it seemed to her, people were pouring in from every corner. She was a novelty to most of our extended relatives, many of whom hadn't met her yet. The idea of personal space in India does not extend to children. Total strangers would come up to her and pinch her cheeks or squeeze her nose. Her pale-white skin was too tempting not to touch, as was her soft light-brown hair, which fell in short ringlets around her face like Shirley Temple's. "You are so cute, Krishna *kutti*," they wailed in their thick accents as they tried to engage her. "Stop touching me!" Krishna wailed back. Krishna was *pissed*. She struggled to find an unpopulated corner of the house. I had to speak to her about respecting her elders, but at three, the cultural differences were hard for her to adapt to.

I wondered then if Krishna would have the same connection to family that I did, with all of us cousins functioning more like siblings. It was the love and support of all these people that had seen me through the various tumults of my life. Suddenly, in the middle of my family, who practically knew me better than I knew myself, I began to miss Teddy terribly. Coming here had been good. It had woken me up from my grief-stricken stupor, but I couldn't shake the feeling that something was missing. It was Teddy. Teddy should have been there with me in that place I considered home. Teddy had shown me so much. Teddy had taught me about unconditional love and forgiveness. I could hear his voice in my head as I looked at the floor trying to find a place to sit. "This is the only game in town, Junior. Big tribe. Everyone should be so lucky."

So when I received a letter from Adam the following Christmas, at the end of 2013, it was Teddy I thought of, of the forgiveness he had shown me, and of the way he had loved Krishna, how he had placed her and my well-being above his own hurt or pain. It had been almost two years since I had taken the stand in the Supreme Court of the State of New York, since Adam and I had reached our custody settlement. Since then he had been a consistent, present, and loving father to Krishna. He had hardly missed a day of his time with her, and I could see how much Krishna had blossomed under the warmth of his love. He took great and enthusiastic care with anything related to her. I didn't spend much time in his company, but I knew my child enough to see that her well-being was also due to him. I tried to focus on that. It was what counted now.

Adam's letter was long: five pages handwritten in his minuscule chicken scrawl, about eight pages in human penmanship. In it he covered many topics. He spoke of his love for Krishna, thanked me for being a good mother, apologized for the lawsuit and for hurting me. And he wrote of how much he enjoyed being a father. I wasn't sure if I believed everything in there, but I didn't doubt for a moment his love for Krishna. The letter softened me. I could appreciate the courage it must have taken to write it.

For two years Adam had tried to get various messages to me through mutual friends. Every once in a while, he invited me for a drink or dinner via text or e-mail. I always declined. In those days, my housekeeper or I would bring Krishna down to the lobby rather than allow Adam up the elevator to come to our front door. His main sources of information about me were Tara's husband, Matt, who knew him well from before, and my mother, who kept in occasional telephonic contact with him. Matt tried to lobby for Adam, feeling that he had changed a lot after becoming a dad. I told Matt that if Adam had anything to say, he should write me a letter, not pass messages as if he were in high school. And so I had received his magnum opus of a letter.

I gingerly answered the letter and thanked him for the olive branch and apologies. But it would take time, I wrote. The following February, in 2014, his mother passed away after a long battle with cancer. I knew Adam was grieving. For some time, Adam had been asking if I would join him and Krishna for dinner at his house. It seemed like a yes from me could be my first olive branch, and that perhaps the three of us being together, even if it was awkward and tentative, might do some small part to ease his grief. I could hardly say no. Krishna was ecstatic to have both her parents in the same room.

After the success of that first dinner, Adam invited me the following month to an Ides of March dinner. He and Krishna were going to make homemade pizzas and dress as Romans in togas. Again, I said yes, remembering how much joy it would bring Krishna. I dressed up in my old Princess Bithia costume from the *Ten Commandments* miniseries I had filmed years before. Adam insisted we had to immortalize the night—

our costumes were just too good not to get a photo of. I sat stiffly, and nervously on the couch, Krishna between us, while his housekeeper took a photo. We all looked quite splendid in our ridiculous family portrait. The Ides of March dinner marked a turning point for Adam and me. It wasn't a 180-degree about-face, more like a gentle bend in the road, but from that point forward, Adam, Krishna, and I had a monthly get-together. We agreed Krishna needed to see her parents get along. We both felt it was important for her to feel we were sharing notes, informing each other of her life, communicating. She was four by then, sharp and keenly observant.

Over the course of that year, we lurched forward bit by bit, month by month. My chill, though not my caution, toward Adam began to thaw. As Christmas approached, Krishna decided she desperately wanted our monthly outing to be ice-skating at Rockefeller Center, followed by seeing the larger-than-life tree (this from a kid with one Hindu and one Jewish parent). Until then, all of our monthly get-togethers had happened in private, so going to Rockefeller Center at the height of the holiday season made me queasy at best.

I had grown up in New York, too, just like Krishna, however different our lives may otherwise have been, and I remembered acutely how special an occasion it was to go ice-skating at Rockefeller Center. My mother could rarely afford it—the skate rentals were so costly. It was a memory I wanted to make with Krishna, as I had made it with my own mother. I couldn't resist and agreed to go.

That chilly Saturday, Krishna and I arrived at Rockefeller Center close to six. We had just gotten out of a matinee of the movie *Annie,* emerging into a dark winter night. Christmas was just around the corner, and Rockefeller Center was bursting with holiday shoppers, out-of-town tourists, and Salvation Army Santas ringing the bells. Glittering wreaths and tinsel garlands adorned the shop fronts, and the display windows were done up to the nines, functioning as elaborate holiday dioramas: toy trains circling miniature tracks that traversed snow-sparkling miniature villages of dazzlingly complex detail. It was hard to find space to maneuver on the sidewalk. I had recently acquired a highly impractical, extremely puffy red goat-hair coat that made the upper half of my body look like a giant cranberry snowball. So it was hard to even carry Krishna in my arms. She was also almost five and getting heavier every day. My baby wasn't really a baby anymore. The air was bitingly cold, so much so that you needed a hat and gloves to be comfortable outside for any length of time. It pricked our faces, though we ignored this by keeping ourselves moving.

The minute I caught sight of the glass elevator at the entrance to Rockefeller Center, I instantly smelled the undeniable aroma of roasting chestnuts, blackened on iron skillets by the seasonal street vendors. The scent had always heralded the holidays for me and my mother. Though ice-skating trips were expensive, and though my mother herself could not ice-skate (she often stood at the edge of the rink and watched me skate alone), part of what we loved about making the excursion were those delicious roasted chestnuts. We loved the earthy smell of them, the acrid whiff of char combined with the sweetness of the nut meat. We relished holding the hot little stones in our hands, then stuffing our pockets with the crinkly paper bags of nuts, which functioned as impromptu hand warmers, pulling out one chestnut at a time and peeling it gingerly, the released steam stinging our naked fingers. We loved the charred, chewy outer parts, and the steaming, soft, almost buttery centers, too. Our Rockefeller Center outings were, actually, almost entirely an excuse to indulge in this wintertime delicacy. Standing there thirty-five years later, the scent instantly transported me to being nine years old again. I wished I could somehow harness the aroma and mail an envelope of it to my mother in California, who was right then probably trimming the roses in her sun-filled front yard.

I looked up at the night sky. High above all the national flags flapping vigorously in the winter wind, as well as the larger-than-life toy soldiers, the great Christmas tree towered above everything, twinkly and imposing. I pointed it out to Krishna, who was far more enchanted with the statue of Prometheus at its base. Below the golden Titan lay the ice rink, shimmering and impossibly white, crowded by holiday revelers crisscrossing it in loops and twirls. We waited there for Adam to meet us and take us to the VIP entrance, which until recently I never even knew existed. Adam had generously paid extra so we would not have to wait in line. He knew about my aversion to crowds, and I appreciated this added luxury.

Adam emerged from the sea of people on the plaza. He was tall and easy to see. He grabbed Krishna and swiftly put her up on his shoulders above the crowd. Her face lit up as bright as the big tree. We waited in line for the elevator, and he put her down as we went in. Once downstairs in the shopping arcade, we went into the small VIP area to get our skates, joining a couple of other families there. Beyond the doors, I saw a steady stream of skaters, all in a bunch, going around and around the rink like a school of fish. How were we going to wade into that? Adam helped Krishna with her tiny little rental skates, and I somehow managed to bend over and get mine on in spite of the puffball coat. A man helping his own daughter and son with their skates smiled at Adam and Krishna and said, "What a lovely child." "Thank you!" Adam and I both responded in unison. We looked at each other and I smiled sheepishly, but also couldn't help but feel territorial. It was a rare and strange occurrence for us to experience the feeling of joint pride.

"You ready, Mommy?" Krishna asked. I nodded silently as Adam led her to the entrance of the rink. He patiently helped her walk on her skates. She looked so small next to him. Beyond their silhouettes, I could see the people, the steady stream of skaters. I hurried and went out ahead, onto the ice first, and held on to the rink wall. I needed some air. The spectators looking down from above made me feel like I was in a Roman amphitheater. A knot of teenagers whizzed by, followed by a young couple holding hands, going slowly and trying to steady themselves. An elderly woman and a young man who looked like her grandson glided by arm in arm. They looked like they had been skating all their lives. I thought then about my future seventy-year-old self, bringing Krishna's son or daughter to this very place my mother had first brought me. There were families of all sorts of sizes and colors. In the middle of the rink twirled skaters who looked almost semiprofessional, dressed in lighter skating costumes, elegant cloth covers over their own skates. They pirouetted and glided with swan-like elegance, and the other, average skaters falling and tripping behind them in the far curve of the rink made for a comical backdrop.

The spirit of the crowd took me out of my own anxiety. Everyone was so happy. Everyone was smiling. But no two smiles were bigger than Krishna's and her dad's. You could see her two little dimples piercing deep into her chin just under her upturned rosy lips, pressed tightly together. Her cheeks looked like they would burst. "You ready, Mommy?" Adam repeated. I took a deep breath. We started out very slowly on the ice, Krishna in the middle, holding each of our hands. Since none of us were that steady, we stayed on the outer perimeter, going very slowly. We were new at this. At all of it. It felt dangerous, like the ice was thin and might break open at any moment to swallow us whole. But the ground did not open up. Ahead of us, I saw a couple of kids tumble and fall, but get up instantly before we reached them. They skated onward like nothing had happened.

I glanced down at Krishna, who was having some trouble staying upright on her skates. But she hung in there, joyful and excited. We went around a few times and got the hang of it, more or less. The three of us managed to stay vertical, as well as dodge those who fell in our path. Little by little, we gained our confidence. We picked up speed, too. This was the challenge we had been working up to all these many months. It felt exhilarating to be gliding on that ice, the three of us together holding hands. I even felt brave enough to let go of Krishna's hand and skate backward briefly, facing Adam and our daughter. Years of skating in the city came back to my legs. The rink was too busy to do it for long, but I was glad I had taken the risk. I asked them if they wanted to stop and take a break. Adam looked at me and smiled. *"No. Are you kidding?"* he said. "I want hot chocolate! I want cookies!" Krishna pleaded. We skated around a bit more and then went back into the rental area for a break. As we sat back in the warmth and had our snacks, I thought about where I would be in my life the next time I came to this rink. Being here had always been a special occasion, a treat to be savored, remembered. On no occasion was this more so than that evening.

The baby was getting older. We had done a pretty good job of maintaining a civil, polite rapport between us in front of her, even through the worst of it. We had been successfully following through on our monthly get-togethers, so Krishna could experience the feeling of having her family together. But it was Adam who had been the driving force behind the idea. The dinners and outings were arranged and coaxed into existence by Adam and Adam alone. I could see he was trying very hard to create a new history for us as friends.

I left Adam and Krishna inside and went to skate by myself, so I could try going faster. After a few rounds, I got my speed up pretty good. I saw Adam and Krishna enter the rink. I sped up enough to go around once and pass them. They tried to catch up, and then, like a pile of dominos, we all fell on top of one another. Krishna and I couldn't stop laughing long enough to get up, and we struggled to stand, our bodies tangled on the ice. Adam got up and extended his hand to help me. Krishna was scrambling around my feet. She looked up toward me. "Mom, take his hand. Let Dad help you."

Family was important to both Adam and me, and I wanted to somehow instill that in Krishna, too. But I could not underline the importance
of family unless I accepted the whole of hers. So rather than be mired in
the ugliness of our past, I came to be propelled forward by our shared love
for her. In a sense, it was the same love and forgiveness Teddy had shown
me, unconditional in the wake of everything that had happened, bound-
less in its generosity. It was easy to follow his example for Krishna's sake. I
am sure Krishna's father had some forgiving to do as well in my regard. If
he had trouble with this, he did not show it, or speak of needing anything
from me to do it.

"Yeah, Mommy; let me help you."

We went back out into the night, the three of us together, skating
hand in hand.

acknowledgments

First of all, my deep gratitude goes to Daniel Halpern, Libby Edelson, and Luke Janklow, without whom I could never have written this book. And to my assistant Tucker Gurley, without whom I would never have gotten through the last several years. Undying thanks also to all my family, especially the women in my clan and most of all to my mother, Vijaya Lakshmi, because my story is also her story, and she has had the courage and grace to let me tell it as I see fit. My thanks also to Krishna's father, Adam Dell. And to Salman for planting the seed so many years ago over tandoori on Lexington Avenue, for being a cheerleader and handing me Rousseau. Thank you to Susan Roxborough for being the kind of friend and in-house editor every writer should have. Thank you to my many recipe testers like Jolie Hunt, Judith Sutton, and my writing assistant Caroline Perkins, as well as to those who read early versions or heard pieces of the book over late nights and many telephone calls, including Sharon Sperling, Kristin Powers, Bonnie Takhar, Jason Comis, Dr. Sylvia Karasu, and so many more. Thank you to JJ Goode for understanding that I had to write this book on my own, a different book than when I started. And much gratitude goes to the late great Nora Ephron for her generous mentorship in the last year of her life, without which this book would not have its title. Thank you finally to my late grandfather, K. C. Krishnamurti, and my beloved grandmother, CVS Rajilakshmi, for instilling in me the love of books and cooking, two things I could not live without.

PADMA LAKSHMI is the Emmy-nominated host of the highly rated and critically acclaimed, Emmy-winning Bravo series *Top Chef,* and the author of two cookbooks: *Tangy, Tart, Hot & Sweet* and the award-winning *Easy Exotic.* In addition to her culinary achievements, Lakshmi has contributed to such magazines as *Vogue, Gourmet,* and *Harper's Bazaar* (UK and US), and penned a syndicated column on fashion and food for the *New York Times.* Her television-hosting credits include *Planet Food* and *Padma's Passport,* as well as other programs in the United States and abroad. A global style icon and the first internationally successful Indian supermodel, Lakshmi also helms companies of her own such as the Padma Collection and Easy Exotic.

Lakshmi is a cofounder of the Endometriosis Foundation of America. Since 2009, the organization has advocated for early diagnosis, promoted research, and raised awareness in the medical community and the greater public about this devastating chronic disease which affects over 190 million women worldwide.

She lives in New York City with her daughter.